WALL PILA
FOR WOMEN
OVER 60

Discover Wall Pilates Techniques and Methods to Strengthen Your Body with Low-Impact Home Workouts for Women and Beginners.

MARY D. BEVERIDGE

Copyright© [2024] by [MARY D. BEVERIDGE]

All rights reserved. No part of this book may be reproduced, distributed, or transmitted in any form or by any means, including photocopying, recording, or other electronic or mechanical methods, without the prior written permission of the publisher, except in the case of brief quotations embodied in critical reviews and certain other noncommercial uses permitted by copyright law.

Table of Contents

Introduction — 5
    Understanding Wall Pilates — 5
    What Is Wall Pilates? — 6
    Benefits for Women Over 60 — 7
    Getting Started Safely — 9

Chapter 1 — 12
    Setting Up Your Home Workout Space — 12
    Necessary Equipment — 15

Chapter 2 — 18
    Warm-Up and Stretching — 18
    Gentle Exercises to Prepare Your Body — 21
    Limbering Up for the Workout — 24

Chapter 3 — 28
    Core Strengthening Wall Pilates — 28
    Building a Solid Foundation — 31
    Targeting Your Core Muscles — 34

Chapter 4 — 38
    Wall Pilates for Flexibility — 38
    Stretching Routines for Suppleness — 41

Chapter 5 — 46
    Strength and Balance — 46

Boosting Muscular Strength	52
Improving Balance and Stability	58

Chapter 6   65

Low-Impact Wall Pilates Workouts	65
Full-Body Workouts	69
Focused Exercises for Different Needs	73
Advancing Your Wall Pilates Practice	81
Taking It to the Next Level	85

Chapter 8   89

Recovery and Self-Care	89
Restorative Practices	93
Self-Care Tips for Women Over 60	97
Building Consistency	100

Conclusion   104

Achieving Your Wellness Goals	104
Embracing a Healthier Lifestyle	108

Bouns   111

30-Day Wall Pilates Workouts Challenge for Women Over 60	111

Introduction

Understanding Wall Pilates

Welcome to the world of Wall Pilates, a unique and empowering fitness method made specifically for women over 60 and beginners. In this chapter, we will delve into the fundamentals of Wall Pilates, helping you grasp the core concepts, benefits, and skills that will guide your journey towards a healthier, stronger, and more flexible you.

Wall Pilates is not just another workout routine; it's a mindful practice that combines elements of traditional Pilates with the support and stability of a wall. It is designed to be gentle on the body while delivering profound results, making it an ideal choice for those looking to enhance their physical well-being in a safe and enjoyable way.

In this chapter, we will see through what Wall Pilates is all about, outlining its origins and principles. You'll discover how this form of exercise can uniquely benefit women over 60, addressing common concerns and providing solutions for improved vitality and strength.

Whether you're completely new to Pilates or have some experience, this chapter will lay the foundation for your Wall Pilates journey. We'll cover essential concepts and terminology, ensuring that you have a solid understanding of the practice before we dive into the routines and workouts that follow.

So, let's embark on this journey of self-discovery and empowerment through Wall Pilates. By the end of this chapter, you'll have a clear understanding of what lies ahead and the confidence to embrace this transformative fitness method. Get ready to strengthen your body, improve your posture, and enhance your overall well-being with Wall Pilates.

What Is Wall Pilates?

Most beginners or people seem to not know what wall Pilates means, Wall Pilates is a specialised form of exercise that combines the principles of traditional Pilates with the support and stability provided by a wall. It focuses on enhancing core strength, flexibility, balance, and overall body awareness. In Wall Pilates, participants use the wall as a prop to perform various exercises, making it an accessible and low-impact fitness option suitable for women over 60 and beginners.

At its core, Wall Pilates emphasizes controlled movements, proper breathing, and alignment, all of which contribute to improved posture and a stronger, more toned body. By using the wall for support, individuals can perform exercises with greater stability and reduced strain on their joints, making it an ideal choice for those seeking a safe and effective fitness routine.

Benefits for Women Over 60

Enhanced Heart Health: Engaging in regular physical activity, such as walking, swimming, or cycling, can help maintain cardiovascular health. It reduces the risk of heart disease and lowers blood pressure, benefiting women over 60 who may be more susceptible to these issues.

Improved Bone Health: Aging can lead to decreased bone density, making bones more fragile and susceptible to fractures. Weight-bearing exercises and strength training can help preserve bone density and reduce the risk of osteoporosis.

Joint Health: Low-impact exercises like yoga is gentle on the joints and can alleviate joint pain and stiffness, common concerns for women in this age group.

Enhanced Flexibility: Stretching exercises can improve flexibility, making daily activities easier and reducing the risk of muscle strains.

Weight Management: Regular physical activity helps maintain a healthy weight, which is essential for overall health and can reduce the risk of obesity-related conditions such as diabetes and certain cancers.

Mental Well-being: Exercise releases endorphins, which can combat feelings of depression and anxiety. Staying active is a powerful tool for maintaining mental health and cognitive function.

Social Engagement: Participating in group activities, whether it's a fitness class or a walking club, can provide social interaction and combat feelings of loneliness and isolation.

Improved Sleep: Regular exercise can contribute to better sleep quality, which is essential for overall health and well-being.

Cognitive Benefits: Physical activity has been linked to improved cognitive function and a reduced risk of cognitive decline in older adults.

Longevity: Leading an active lifestyle has been associated with a longer and more fulfilling life. Regular exercise can increase life expectancy and improve the quality of those extra years.

Reduced Chronic Disease Risk: Physical activity can reduce the risk of chronic diseases such as type 2 diabetes, certain cancers, and stroke, helping women in this age group maintain their health.

Maintaining physical fitness can help women over 60 maintain their independence by ensuring they can perform daily tasks and activities without the help of an assistance.

Incorporating a well-rounded exercise routine into your daily life can bring about these numerous benefits, contributing to a healthier and more enjoyable journey through your 60s and beyond.

Getting Started Safely

Embarking on a fitness journey, especially if you're new to exercise or haven't been active for a while, requires careful consideration of safety. This is particularly important for women over 60, as your body may have specific needs and limitations. Here are some essential tips to ensure you get started safely:

1. Consult Your Healthcare Provider: Before beginning any exercise program, consult with your healthcare provider, especially if you have pre-existing medical conditions or concerns. They can provide valuable guidance on what types of activities are safe and appropriate for you.

2. Set Realistic Goals: Start with realistic and achievable fitness goals. Whether it's increasing daily steps, improving flexibility, or building strength, setting attainable objectives will keep you motivated and prevent overexertion.

3. Warm-Up and Cool Down: Prior to each workout, dedicate time to warm-up exercises to prepare your muscles and joints. Afterward, engage in a cool-down routine to help your body recover gradually.

4. Stay Hydrated: Adequate hydration is essential, especially as we age. Drink water before, during, and after your workouts to prevent dehydration.

5. Proper Footwear: Invest in supportive and comfortable footwear appropriate for your

chosen activities. Proper shoes can reduce the risk of falls and injuries.

6. Balance Exercises: Incorporate balance exercises into your routine to improve stability and reduce the risk of falls. Activities like tai chi or yoga can be beneficial.

7. Listen to Your Body: Pay close attention to how your body feels during exercise. If you experience pain, dizziness, or extreme discomfort, stop immediately and seek medical advice if necessary.

8. Variety is Key: Include a variety of activities in your fitness routine to work different muscle groups and prevent boredom. This can also reduce the risk of overuse injuries.

By prioritizing safety and taking a gradual approach to exercise, you can enjoy the numerous benefits of physical activity while minimizing the risk of injuries or setbacks. Remember that consistency and patience are key to long-term success on your fitness journey.

Chapter 1

Setting Up Your Home Workout Space

Creating a conducive and comfortable workout space at home is an essential step in establishing a successful fitness routine, especially for women over 60. A well-organized workout area ensures you have the motivation, convenience, and safety needed to stay committed to your exercise goals. Here are some tips on setting up your home workout space:

1. Choose the Right Location: Select a dedicated area in your home where you can exercise without interruptions. Ideally, this space should be well-ventilated and well-lit. Natural light can be particularly motivating.

2. Clear the Clutter: Declutter the chosen space to create a clean and open environment. Remove any obstacles or hazards that could pose a tripping or safety risk.

3. Invest in a Quality Mat: A high-quality exercise mat provides comfort and support for floor exercises. Look for one that is thick enough to cushion your joints and non-slip to prevent accidents.

4. Use Proper Lighting: Adequate lighting is crucial for safety and visibility during your workouts. Consider installing extra lighting or using portable lamps to brighten the area.

5. Mirror, Mirror: If possible, place a full-length mirror in your workout space. A mirror helps you monitor your form and technique, which is particularly important for exercises like yoga and Pilates.

6. Storage Solutions: Organize your workout equipment neatly. Shelving, bins, or cabinets can help keep weights, resistance bands, and other gear organized and easily accessible.

7. Technology Setup: If you follow online workout videos or use fitness apps, ensure your home workout space has access to a screen (TV, tablet, or smartphone) and a stable internet connection.

8. Ventilation and Climate Control: Ensure your workout area is well-ventilated, and consider

climate control options like fans or heaters to maintain a comfortable temperature.

9. Safety Measures: Install safety equipment if necessary, such as handrails or grab bars for stability, especially if you're doing exercises that involve balance.

10. Personal Touch: Add elements that motivate and inspire you. This could be posters of fitness quotes, calming artwork, or anything that creates a positive atmosphere.

11. Music and Audio: Set up a music system or speakers to play your favorite workout tunes or calming background music, depending on your preference.

12. Privacy and Distraction-Free: Inform your household about your workout schedule to minimize distractions. Let them know when you prefer uninterrupted exercise time.

13. Hydration Station: Have a water source nearby, whether it's a water bottle, a dispenser, or a small fridge stocked with cold water to keep you hydrated during workouts.

By creating a dedicated and inviting home workout space, you'll remove common barriers to exercise and make it more likely that you'll stick to your fitness routine. Your home gym can become a sanctuary for wellness and personal growth as you progress on your fitness journey.

Necessary Equipment

Wall Pilates is a versatile and accessible form of exercise that requires minimal equipment, making it well-suited for women over 60. Here's a list of the necessary equipment to get started with Wall Pilates:

1. Wall Space: As the name suggests, you'll need access to a sturdy wall. Ensure it's clean, dry, and free from obstructions. A smooth, flat surface is ideal for a comfortable practice.

2. Exercise Mat: A high-quality exercise mat provides cushioning and support for floor exercises, enhancing your comfort and safety.

3. Comfortable Clothing: Wear comfortable and breathable workout attire that allows for freedom of movement. Choose moisture-wicking fabrics to keep you dry during exercise.

4. Footwear: For many Wall Pilates exercises, you can go barefoot or wear grippy socks with non-slip soles. These provide traction and stability when moving along the wall.

5. Resistance Bands: Resistance bands are versatile tools that can be used to add resistance and intensity to your Wall Pilates exercises. They come in various levels of resistance, so choose bands that suit your fitness level.

6. Yoga Blocks: Yoga blocks can be helpful for modifying exercises or providing support during stretches. They can assist with balance and flexibility.

7. Small Pillow or Cushion: A small pillow or cushion can provide extra support for your head or lower back during certain exercises.

8. Water Bottle: Staying hydrated during your workout is essential. Keep a water bottle nearby to sip on as needed.

9. Mirror: While not mandatory, having a full-length mirror in your workout space can be beneficial for checking your form and alignment during exercises.

10. Timer or Stopwatch: Having a timer or stopwatch can help you keep track of exercise durations and rest intervals, ensuring you follow your workout plan effectively.

11. Chair or Wall-Mounted Bar: Depending on your needs and the exercises you perform, a sturdy chair or a wall-mounted bar can be used for additional support during certain Wall Pilates movements.

12. Music or Audio Device: Consider using a music player or audio device to play your favorite workout music or follow along with instructional audio cues.

13. Exercise Ball (Optional): Some Wall Pilates variations may incorporate an exercise ball for added challenge and variety. It's not necessary for all exercises, but it can be a useful addition.

These items are the basic equipment needed to start your Wall Pilates journey. As you progress and become more familiar with the practice, you may choose to explore additional props and equipment to diversify your workouts further. However, for beginners and women over 60, this list provides a solid foundation for a safe and effective Wall Pilates routine.

Chapter 2

Warm-Up and Stretching

A proper warm-up and stretching routine is a crucial part of any fitness regimen, especially for women over 60. These preparatory exercises not only help prevent injury but also enhance your overall workout experience. Here's a tailored warm-up and stretching routine designed with your specific needs in mind:

Warm-Up (5-10 minutes):

1. March in Place: Begin by marching in place for a few minutes. This gentle movement raises your heart rate and warms up your leg muscles.

2. Arm Circles: Stand with your feet hip-width apart and extend your arms straight out to the sides. Make small circles with your arms, gradually increasing their size. Repeat for 30 seconds in each direction.

3. Torso Twists: With your feet shoulder-width apart, place your hands on your hips. Slowly twist your torso to the right, then back to center, and then to the left. Continue this motion for 30 seconds.

4. Knee Lifts: Stand with your feet hip-width apart. Lift your right knee towards your chest, then lower it. Alternate between your right and left knees for 30 seconds.

5. Ankle Circles: Sit on a chair or stand with one foot slightly off the ground. Rotate your ankle in a circular motion for 15 seconds in each direction. Repeat with the other ankle.

Stretching (5-10 minutes):

1. Neck Stretch: Gently tilt your head to the right, bringing your right ear towards your right shoulder. Hold for 15 seconds, then switch to the left side.

2. Shoulder Rolls: Roll your shoulders forward and backward in a slow, circular motion. Repeat for 30 seconds in each direction.

3. Chest Opener: Interlace your fingers behind your back and straighten your arms. Lift your arms slightly and open your chest, squeezing your shoulder blades together. Hold for 15 seconds.

4. Arm Across Body Stretch: Extend your right arm in front of you and bring it across your chest. Use your left hand to gently press your right arm closer

to your chest. Hold for 15 seconds, then switch sides.

5. Standing Quadriceps Stretch: Hold onto a wall or a chair for balance. Bend your right knee, bringing your heel towards your buttocks. Hold your ankle with your right hand and gently pull to feel a stretch in your quadriceps. Hold for 15 seconds, then switch legs.

6. Calf Stretch: Stand facing a wall with one foot in front of the other. Lean forward slightly, keeping your back leg straight and your heel on the ground. You should feel a stretch in your calf muscle. Hold for 15 seconds on each leg.

7. Standing Hamstring Stretch: Stand with your feet hip-width apart. Take a step forward with your right foot and bend your right knee slightly. Keep your left leg straight and bend forward from your hips, reaching towards your right foot. Hold for 15 seconds, then switch sides.

8. Seated Forward Bend: Sit on a chair with your feet flat on the ground. Extend your arms forward and slowly hinge at your hips, leaning your torso forward. Reach as far as is comfortable while keeping your back straight. Hold for 15 seconds.

This warm-up and stretching routine is designed to prepare your body for Wall Pilates exercises while promoting flexibility and reducing the risk of injury. Always perform these exercises at a comfortable pace, and if you experience pain or discomfort, modify them to suit your needs.

Gentle Exercises to Prepare Your Body

Before diving into more intensive Wall Pilates exercises, it's important to engage in gentle movements that prepare your body and awaken your muscles. These exercises are specifically tailored for women over 60 to ensure a safe and effective warm-up:

1. Neck Tilts (Neck Mobility):
   - Sit or stand with your back straight.
   - Slowly tilt your head to the right, bringing your right ear towards your right shoulder.
   - Hold for a few seconds, feeling a gentle stretch along the left side of your neck.
   - Return your head to the center and repeat on the left side.
   - Perform 5-10 repetitions on each side.

2. Shoulder Rolls (Shoulder Mobility):
   - Stand or sit comfortably with your arms at your sides.
   - Slowly roll your shoulders forward in a circular motion.
   - After 10-15 seconds, reverse the direction and roll your shoulders backward.
   - Perform 2-3 sets of 10-15 seconds in each direction.

3. Arm Swings (Arm Mobility):
   - Stand with your feet shoulder-width apart.
   - Extend your arms out to the sides.
   - Swing your arms forward and then backward in a controlled manner.
   - Perform this exercise for 30 seconds, gradually increasing the range of motion.

4. Ankle Circles (Ankle Mobility):
   - Sit on a chair or stand with one foot slightly off the ground.
   - Rotate your ankle in a circular motion for 15 seconds in one direction.
   - Reverse the direction and continue for another 15 seconds.
   - Switch to the other ankle and repeat.

5. Gentle Leg Lifts (Leg Mobility):

- Stand behind a sturdy chair or use a wall for support.
- Hold onto the chair or wall for balance.
- Lift one leg straight out in front of you, keeping your knee extended but not locked.
- Lower the leg back down and repeat with the other leg.
- Perform 5-10 repetitions on each leg.

6. Deep Breathing (Diaphragmatic Breathing):
   - Sit or lie down in a comfortable position.
   - Place one hand on your chest and the other on your abdomen.
   - Inhale deeply through your nose, allowing your abdomen to rise as you fill your lungs.
   - Exhale slowly through your mouth, feeling your abdomen fal.
   - Repeat this deep breathing exercise for 1-2 minutes to relax and center yourself.

These gentle exercises are designed to gradually increase blood flow, warm up your muscles, and improve joint mobility. They are an excellent way to prepare your body for more challenging Wall Pilates movements and ensure a safe and enjoyable workout experience. Always listen to your body, and if any exercise causes pain or discomfort, stop and consult with a healthcare professional.

Limbering Up for the Workout

Limbering up your body is a crucial step to ensure that you're ready for your Wall Pilates workout. These gentle movements and stretches will help increase blood flow, improve flexibility, and prepare your muscles for more intense exercises. Here's a limbering up routine designed for women over 60:

1. Gentle Neck Tilts (Neck Mobility):
    - Sit or stand with your back straight.
    - Slowly tilt your head to the right, bringing your right ear toward your right shoulder.
    - Hold for a few seconds, feeling a gentle stretch along the left side of your neck.
    - Return your head to the center and repeat on the left side.
    - Perform 5-10 repetitions on each side.

2. Shoulder Rolls (Shoulder Mobility):
    - Stand or sit comfortably with your arms at your sides.
    - Slowly roll your shoulders forward in a circular motion.
    - After 10-15 seconds, reverse the direction and roll your shoulders backward.
    - Perform 2-3 sets of 10-15 seconds in each direction.

3. Arm Swings (Arm Mobility):
    - Stand with your feet shoulder-width apart.
    - Extend your arms out to the sides.
    - Swing your arms forward and then backward in a controlled manner.
    - Perform this exercise for 30 seconds, gradually increasing the range of motion.

4. Side Bends (Torso Mobility):
    - Stand with your feet hip-width apart, arms at your sides.
    - Slowly bend your upper body to the right, keeping your feet planted.
    - Return to the center and then bend to the left.
    - Perform 5-10 repetitions on each side.

5. Hip Circles (Hip Mobility):
    - Stand with your feet hip-width apart, hands on your hips.
    - Slowly circle your hips clockwise for 15 seconds.
    - Reverse the direction and circle your hips counterclockwise for another 15 seconds.

6. Knee Lifts (Leg Mobility):
    - Stand behind a sturdy chair or use a wall for support.
    - Hold onto the chair or wall for balance.

- Lift one knee toward your chest while keeping your back straight.
- Lower the leg back down and repeat with the other leg.
- Perform 5-10 repetitions on each leg.

7. Ankle Circles (Ankle Mobility):
    - Sit on a chair or stand with one foot slightly off the ground.
    - Rotate your ankle in a circular motion for 15 seconds in one direction.
    - Reverse the direction and continue for another 15 seconds.
    - Switch to the other ankle and repeat.

8. Deep Breathing (Diaphragmatic Breathing):
    - Sit or lie down in a comfortable position.
    - Place one hand on your chest and the other on your abdomen.
    - Inhale deeply through your nose, allowing your abdomen to rise as you fill your lungs.
    - Exhale slowly through your mouth, feeling your abdomen fall.
    - Repeat this deep breathing exercise for 1-2 minutes to relax and center yourself.

Limbering up with these gentle exercises will help you ease into your Wall Pilates workout, reducing the risk of strain or injury while enhancing your overall mobility and comfort during the session. Always perform these exercises at a comfortable pace and within your range of motion.

Chapter 3

Core Strengthening Wall Pilates

Building a strong and stable core is essential for women over 60, as it not only supports good posture but also contributes to overall balance and functional fitness. Wall Pilates offers an effective and low-impact way to target and strengthen your core muscles. Here's a guide to core-strengthening Wall Pilates exercises tailored for women over 60:

1. Wall Squats with Core Engagement:
   - Stand with your back against the wall and your feet hip-width apart.
   - Slowly lower your body into a squat position while keeping your back against the wall.
   - As you rise back up, engage your core muscles by pulling your navel toward your spine.
   - Perform 10-12 repetitions.

2. Wall Planks:
   - Stand facing the wall about an arm's length away.
   - Place your hands on the wall at shoulder height, shoulder-width apart.

- Step your feet back and extend your body into a plank position.
- Keep your core engaged, and your body in a straight line from head to heels.
- Hold the plank for 20-30 seconds, gradually increasing the duration as you become stronger.

3. Leg Lifts with Wall Support:
   - Stand facing the wall, placing your hands on the wall for support.
   - Lift your right leg straight back and up, engaging your glutes and core.
   - Lower your leg back down and repeat on the left side.
   - Perform 10-12 repetitions on each leg.

4. Wall Bridge:
   - Lie on your back with your feet flat on the wall and your knees bent.
   - Place your arms at your sides.
   - Press through your feet to lift your hips off the floor, creating a bridge shape.
   - Engage your core and squeeze your glutes at the top.
   - Lower your hips back down and repeat for 10-12 repetitions.

5. Wall Sit with Rotation:

- Stand with your back against the wall, feet hip-width apart.
- Lower your body into a wall sit position, thighs parallel to the floor.
- Place your hands together at chest height.
- Rotate your torso to the right, bringing your hands toward the right side of your body.
- Return to the center and then rotate to the left.
- Perform 10-12 repetitions on each side.

6. Wall Teaser (Advanced):
- Sit on the floor with your back against the wall and your knees bent.
- Lift your feet off the ground and straighten your legs, forming a "V" shape.
- Hold this position for a few seconds, engaging your core.
- Lower your feet back down and repeat for 5-7 repetitions.

Remember to perform these exercises with proper form and controlled movements. Start with a comfortable number of repetitions and gradually increase as your strength improves. Incorporating these core-strengthening Wall Pilates exercises into your routine can help you maintain a strong and resilient core, supporting your overall health and well-being.

Building a Solid Foundation

As women age, it becomes increasingly important to focus on building a solid foundation of health and well-being. This foundation provides the support needed to lead an active and fulfilling life in your 60s and beyond. Here are key elements to consider when building a solid foundation for women over 60:

1. Regular Exercise: Engaging in regular physical activity is vital for maintaining strength, flexibility, and overall health. Consider low-impact exercises like walking, swimming, yoga, or Wall Pilates to keep your body active and mobile.

2. Balanced Nutrition: A well-balanced diet rich in fruits, vegetables, whole grains, lean proteins, and healthy fats provides essential nutrients for energy, vitality, and disease prevention. Consult with a healthcare professional or nutritionist for personalized dietary recommendations.

3. Adequate Hydration: Staying properly hydrated is essential for various bodily functions. Aim to drink plenty of water throughout the day to support your overall health.

4. Quality Sleep: Prioritize restorative sleep by maintaining a consistent sleep schedule and creating a comfortable sleeping environment. Quality sleep is crucial for physical and mental well-being.

5. Stress Management: Develop effective stress management techniques such as deep breathing exercises, meditation, mindfulness, or engaging in hobbies that bring joy and relaxation.

6. Regular Health Screenings: Schedule regular check-ups and health screenings with your healthcare provider to monitor and manage any underlying health conditions.

7. Social Connections: Maintain an active social life to foster emotional well-being. Connecting with friends, family, or participating in group activities can reduce feelings of loneliness and isolation.

8. Mental Stimulation: Keep your mind sharp through activities like puzzles, reading, learning new skills, or engaging in creative pursuits. Mental stimulation is essential for cognitive health.

9. Bone Health: Focus on bone health by ensuring an adequate intake of calcium and vitamin D, along

with weight-bearing exercises to help prevent osteoporosis and fractures.

10. Flexibility and Mobility: Incorporate stretching exercises and mobility routines into your daily life to maintain joint flexibility and reduce the risk of injury.

11. Emotional Well-Being: Prioritize your emotional health by seeking support when needed, expressing your feelings, and practicing self-compassion.

12. Preventive Care: Stay up-to-date with vaccinations and preventive health measures, as recommended by your healthcare provider.

13. Financial Planning: Plan for your financial future to ensure security and peace of mind as you age. Consult with a financial advisor to make informed decisions.

Building a solid foundation for women over 60 involves a holistic approach to health and well-being. By addressing these key aspects of your life, you can create a strong foundation that supports you in enjoying a fulfilling and active lifestyle in your later years. Remember that it's never too late to invest in your health and well-being.

Targeting Your Core Muscles

A strong and stable core is essential for women over 60 as it contributes to overall strength, balance, and posture. Targeting your core muscles can improve your daily functionality and reduce the risk of injury. Here are some effective core exercises tailored for women over 60:

1. Wall Pilates for Core Strength:
    - Stand facing the wall with your feet hip-width apart.
    - Place your hands on the wall at shoulder height.
    - Engage your core and slowly slide your hands up the wall while maintaining a straight body.
    - Once your arms are fully extended, hold for a few seconds, and then return to the starting position.
    - Perform 10-12 repetitions.

2. Seated Leg Lifts with Wall Support:
    - Sit on a chair with your back straight and feet flat on the floor.

- Place your hands on the sides of the chair for support.
- Lift one leg straight out in front of you, engaging your core.
- Hold for a few seconds, then lower your leg and repeat with the other leg.
- Perform 10-12 repetitions on each leg.

3. Bridge Exercise:
    - Lie on your back with your knees bent and feet flat on the floor.
    - Place your arms at your sides.
    - Lift your hips off the ground while engaging your core and squeezing your glutes.
    - Hold the bridge position for a few seconds, then lower your hips back down.
    - Perform 10-12 repetitions.

4. Standing Side Leg Raises:
    - Stand next to a wall or a sturdy piece of furniture for support.
    - Lift one leg out to the side, keeping it straight and engaging your core.
    - Hold for a few seconds, then lower your leg and repeat on the other side.
    - Perform 10-12 repetitions on each leg.

5. Plank Against the Wall:

- Stand facing the wall about an arm's length away.
- Place your hands on the wall at shoulder height, shoulder-width apart.
- Step your feet back and extend your body into a plank position.
- Keep your core engaged and hold the plank for 20-30 seconds.
- Gradually increase the duration as you become stronger.

6. Standing Oblique Twists:
    - Stand with your feet hip-width apart.
    - Place your hands on your hips.
    - Twist your torso to the right, then back to the center, and then to the left.
    - Perform 10-12 repetitions on each side.

7. Wall Teaser (Advanced):
    - Sit on the floor with your back against the wall, knees bent.
    - Lift your feet off the ground and straighten your legs, forming a "V" shape.
    - Hold this position for a few seconds, engaging your core.
    - Lower your feet back down and repeat for 5-7 repetitions.

These core exercises are designed to be gentle yet effective for women over 60. Incorporate them into your regular fitness routine to strengthen your core muscles, improve your stability, and enhance your overall quality of life. Always perform exercises with proper form and listen to your body's cues. If you have any underlying health conditions, consult with a healthcare professional before starting a new exercise program.

Chapter 4

Wall Pilates for Flexibility

Maintaining flexibility is crucial for women over 60 to enhance mobility, prevent injuries, and promote overall well-being. Wall Pilates offers a gentle and effective way to improve flexibility while also building strength. Here's a series of Wall Pilates exercises tailored for flexibility:

1. Wall-Assisted Leg Stretch:
    - Stand with your side facing the wall, about an arm's length away.
    - Place your inside hand on the wall for support.
    - Lift your outside leg and rest your foot against the wall at hip height.
    - Gently push your leg into the wall, feeling a stretch along your hamstring.
    - Hold the stretch for 15-20 seconds and switch to the other leg.
    - Perform 2-3 stretches on each leg.

2. Wall Calf Stretch:
    - Stand facing the wall and place your hands on the wall for support.

- Step one foot back, keeping it straight with your heel on the ground.
- Bend your front knee slightly, feeling a stretch in your calf.
- Hold for 15-20 seconds and switch to the other leg.
- Perform 2-3 stretches on each leg.

3. Wall Hip Flexor Stretch:
   - Face the wall and place both hands on it for support.
   - Step one foot back into a lunge position, keeping your back leg straight.
   - Bend your front knee and lower your hips slightly to feel a stretch in your hip flexor.
   - Hold for 15-20 seconds and switch to the other leg.
   - Perform 2-3 stretches on each leg.

4. Wall-Assisted Chest Opener:
   - Stand with your back to the wall.
   - Extend your arms straight back and place your hands against the wall at shoulder height.
   - Gently press your chest forward and upward, feeling a stretch in your chest and shoulders.
   - Hold for 15-20 seconds, maintaining good posture.

5. Wall Spinal Twist:
   - Stand facing the wall with your feet hip-width apart.
   - Place your hands on the wall at shoulder height.
   - Slowly twist your torso to one side, keeping your feet planted.
   - Hold the twist for 15-20 seconds, then return to the center and repeat on the other side.

6. Wall-Assisted Quadriceps Stretch:
   - Stand facing the wall and place one hand on it for support.
   - Bend one knee and bring your heel toward your buttocks, grasping your ankle with your free hand.
   - Gently pull your heel closer to your buttocks, feeling a stretch in your quadriceps.
   - Hold for 15-20 seconds on each leg.

7. Wall Shoulder Stretch:
   - Stand with your side facing the wall, about an arm's length away.
   - Extend your arm straight out and place your palm against the wall.
   - Slowly rotate your body away from your arm, feeling a stretch in your shoulder.

- Hold for 15-20 seconds and switch to the other arm.
- Perform 2-3 stretches on each arm.

These Wall Pilates flexibility exercises are designed to be safe and effective for women over 60. Incorporate them into your regular routine to improve your range of motion and maintain flexibility as you age. Always perform stretches gently and within your comfort zone to avoid overstretching or causing discomfort.

Stretching Routines for Suppleness

Stretching is a valuable practice for maintaining suppleness, flexibility, and overall mobility as women age. These stretching routines are specifically tailored for women over 60 to help improve flexibility and reduce the risk of muscle stiffness and injury. Perform each stretch slowly and gently, holding each one for 15-30 seconds. Remember to breathe deeply and comfortably during each stretch. If you experience pain or discomfort, stop immediately.

1. Neck Stretch:
    - Sit or stand with your back straight.

- Slowly tilt your head to the right, bringing your right ear towards your right shoulder.
- Hold for 15-30 seconds, then switch to the left side.
- Repeat 2-3 times on each side.

2. Shoulder Stretch:
    - Stand with your feet shoulder-width apart.
    - Reach your right arm across your chest.
    - Use your left hand to gently pull your right arm closer to your chest.
    - Hold for 15-30 seconds, then switch to the left arm.
    - Repeat 2-3 times on each side.

3. Chest Opener:
    - Stand with your feet hip-width apart.
    - Clasp your hands behind your back and straighten your arms.
    - Lift your arms slightly, opening your chest and squeezing your shoulder blades together.
    - Hold for 15-30 seconds.

4. Standing Quadriceps Stretch:
    - Stand with your feet hip-width apart.
    - Bend your right knee and bring your heel towards your buttocks.
    - Hold your right ankle with your right hand, gently pulling it closer to your buttocks.

- Keep your knees close together and maintain balance.
- Hold for 15-30 seconds on each leg.

5. Hamstring Stretch:
    - Sit on a chair with your feet flat on the floor.
    - Extend your right leg straight out in front of you.
    - Flex your right foot and lean forward slightly from your hips.
    - Reach for your right toes with both hands, feeling a stretch in your hamstring.
    - Hold for 15-30 seconds, then switch to the left leg.
    - Repeat 2-3 times on each leg.

6. Standing Calf Stretch:
    - Stand facing a wall, about an arm's length away.
    - Place both hands on the wall at shoulder height.
    - Step one foot back, keeping it straight with your heel on the ground.
    - Bend your front knee and lean forward, feeling a stretch in your calf.
    - Hold for 15-30 seconds on each leg.

7. Hip Flexor Stretch:

- Kneel on the floor with one knee bent at a 90-degree angle.
- Step your opposite foot forward.
- Shift your weight slightly forward, feeling a stretch in the front of your hip on the bent knee side.
- Hold for 15-30 seconds on each leg.

8. Seated Forward Bend:
   - Sit on the floor with your legs extended straight in front of you.
   - Hinge forward from your hips, reaching for your toes.
   - Keep your back straight and bend from your hips rather than your lower back.
   - Hold for 15-30 seconds.

9. Spinal Twist:
   - Sit on a chair with your feet flat on the floor.
   - Cross your right leg over your left thigh.
   - Twist your upper body to the right, placing your left hand on your right knee.
   - Gently twist and look over your right shoulder.
   - Hold for 15-30 seconds on each side.

10. Ankle Circles:
    - Sit on a chair or stand with one foot slightly off the ground.

- Rotate your ankle in a circular motion for 15 seconds in one direction.
- Reverse the direction and continue for another 15 seconds.
- Switch to the other ankle and repeat.

Incorporate these stretching routines into your daily or weekly routine to maintain suppleness and flexibility. Regular stretching can help improve posture, reduce muscle tension, and promote a greater sense of well-being as you navigate life beyond 60.

Chapter 5

Strength and Balance

Strength and balance are two essential components of overall well-being, especially as we age. For women over 60, focusing on building strength and improving balance is not only crucial for maintaining independence but also for reducing the risk of falls and injuries. In this comprehensive guide, we'll explore the importance of strength and balance, the benefits of incorporating these elements into your life, and practical ways to achieve and maintain them.

The Importance of Strength and Balance

Strength and balance are cornerstones of physical fitness that play a vital role in daily life. Here's why they are particularly significant for women over 60:

1. Independence: Maintaining strength and balance allows you to continue performing daily tasks with ease. This includes activities like walking, carrying groceries, climbing stairs, and even getting up from a chair or sofa.

2. Fall Prevention: As we age, the risk of falls increases. Falls can result in serious injuries, including fractures and head trauma. Improving balance and strength can significantly reduce the risk of falls.

3. Bone Health: Strength training helps maintain bone density, reducing the risk of osteoporosis and fractures, which are more common in older adults.

4. Joint Health: Strong muscles provide support to your joints, reducing the risk of joint pain and arthritis.

5. Confidence and Mental Well-being: Feeling physically capable can boost your confidence and contribute to a positive outlook on life.

Benefits of Strength Training

Strength training, also known as resistance or weight training, involves exercises that work your muscles against resistance. Here are some key benefits for women over 60:

1. Increased Muscle Mass: Strength training can help preserve and build muscle mass, which naturally declines with age.

2. Improved Metabolism: Building muscle can boost your metabolism, helping with weight management and energy levels.

3. Enhanced Bone Health: Resistance exercises promote bone density, reducing the risk of osteoporosis.

4. Better Joint Health: Strong muscles provide better joint support and reduce the risk of joint pain.

5. Functional Fitness: Strength training enhances your ability to perform everyday tasks, improving your overall quality of life.

Benefits of Balance Training

Balance training focuses on improving stability and preventing falls. Here's why it's crucial for women over 60:

1. Fall Prevention: Balance exercises help improve your ability to maintain stability, reducing the risk of falls and related injuries.

2. Better Posture: Improved balance leads to better posture, reducing the risk of musculoskeletal issues and back pain.

3. Enhanced Coordination: Balance training enhances coordination and agility, making everyday movements smoother and more controlled.

4. Increased Confidence: As your balance improves, you'll feel more confident in various situations, both physically and mentally.

5. Cognitive Benefits: Some research suggests that balance training may have cognitive benefits, helping to sharpen your mind.

Practical Tips for Building Strength and Balance

Now that we've established the importance and benefits of strength and balance, let's explore practical ways to incorporate them into your life:

1. Consult a Professional: Before starting any new exercise program, consult with a healthcare provider or fitness professional, especially if you have pre-existing medical conditions or concerns.

2. Strength Training: Include resistance exercises in your routine 2-3 times a week. You can use dumbbells, resistance bands, or bodyweight exercises. Focus on all major muscle groups, including legs, arms, back, chest, and core.

3. Balance Training: Incorporate balance exercises into your routine, such as standing on one foot, walking heel-to-toe, or trying yoga or tai chi. Start with exercises that match your current abilities and gradually progress.

4. Cardiovascular Exercise: Don't forget cardiovascular exercise like walking, swimming, or cycling. It complements strength and balance training and promotes overall heart health.

5. Proper Nutrition:* Support your efforts with a balanced diet rich in nutrients and adequate protein to fuel muscle growth and repair.

6. Hydration: Stay hydrated, as proper hydration is essential for muscle function and overall well-being.

7. Rest and Recovery: Allow your body time to rest and recover between exercise sessions to prevent overtraining and reduce the risk of injury.

8. Stay Consistent: Consistency is key. Set achievable goals and establish a regular exercise routine that you enjoy and can maintain long-term.

9. Seek Professional Guidance: Consider working with a certified personal trainer or physical

therapist, especially if you're new to strength and balance training. They can create a tailored program and provide guidance on proper form and technique.

10. Safety First: Pay attention to safety precautions. Ensure your exercise space is well-lit, free from hazards, and equipped with sturdy handrails if needed.

Sample Strength and Balance Exercises

Here are some sample exercises to get you started:

Strength Exercises:
 - Squats
 - Lunges
 - Push-ups (modified if needed)
 - Dumbbell rows
 - Planks

Balance Exercises:
- Single-leg balance: Stand on one foot with eyes open and then closed.
- Heel-to-toe walk: Walk in a straight line with one foot in front of the other.
- Yoga poses: Try tree pose, warrior pose, or chair pose.

- Tai Chi movements: Gentle flowing movements that promote balance and coordination.

Remember to start slowly and progress at your own pace. If you're uncertain about how to perform these exercises safely, consider seeking guidance from a fitness professional.

Strength and balance are invaluable assets for women over 60. They not only support your daily activities and independence but also contribute to your overall quality of life. By incorporating strength and balance training into your routine, maintaining proper nutrition, and staying consistent, you can enjoy the physical and mental benefits that come with improved strength and stability. Always prioritize safety, consult with professionals as needed, and celebrate your progress along the way to a healthier, more vibrant you.

Boosting Muscular Strength

Muscular strength is the foundation of physical fitness, and it becomes increasingly important as women age, especially for those over 60. Building and maintaining muscular strength can enhance daily life, promote independence, reduce the risk of injury, and contribute to overall well-being. In this explanation, we'll delve into the significance of boosting muscular strength, the benefits it offers, and practical ways to achieve it for women over 60.

The Importance of Muscular Strength

Muscular strength refers to the maximum amount of force your muscles can exert against resistance. This strength plays a crucial role in various aspects of your life, including:

1. Functional Independence: Muscular strength is essential for performing everyday tasks like lifting groceries, getting in and out of chairs, and carrying objects.

2. Fall Prevention: Strong muscles help stabilize your body, reducing the risk of falls and related injuries, which are more common in older adults.

3. Bone Health: Engaging in strength-building exercises supports bone density, reducing the risk of osteoporosis and fractures.

4. Weight Management: Muscle tissue burns more calories at rest than fat tissue, which can aid in weight management and metabolic health.

5. Joint Support: Strong muscles provide support to your joints, reducing the risk of joint pain and arthritis.

6. Improved Posture: Strengthening the muscles that support your spine and core can lead to better posture, reducing the risk of musculoskeletal issues.

Benefits of Boosting Muscular Strength

For women over 60, there are several notable benefits to increasing muscular strength:

1. Enhanced Independence: Strong muscles enable you to maintain independence and perform daily activities with greater ease.

2. Injury Prevention: A stronger body is more resilient and less prone to injury, particularly during falls or accidents.

3. Better Balance: Building leg and core strength can improve balance, reducing the risk of slips and falls.

4. Improved Bone Density: Resistance training helps maintain or increase bone density, reducing the risk of fractures associated with osteoporosis.

5. Functional Fitness: Increased strength makes it easier to engage in hobbies, travel, and participate in social activities.

6. Confidence and Mental Well-being: Feeling physically capable can boost self-confidence and contribute to a positive outlook on life.

Practical Ways to Boost Muscular Strength

Here are some practical steps and considerations for women over 60 to boost muscular strength:

1. Consult a Professional: Before starting any new exercise program, consult with a healthcare provider or fitness professional, especially if you have pre-existing medical conditions or concerns.

2. Resistance Training: Incorporate resistance or strength training exercises into your routine 2-3 times a week. You can use various forms of resistance, including dumbbells, resistance bands, or even your body weight.

3. Target Major Muscle Groups: Focus on all major muscle groups, including legs, arms, back, chest, and core. A well-rounded routine ensures balanced strength development.

4. Proper Form and Technique: Pay close attention to proper form and technique to avoid injury. If you're unsure, consider working with a certified personal trainer.

5. Gradual Progression: Start with a weight or resistance level that is manageable and gradually increase it as your strength improves.

6. Variety: Include a variety of exercises to prevent boredom and target different muscle groups.

7. Rest and Recovery: Allow your muscles time to rest and recover between strength training sessions to promote muscle growth and reduce the risk of overtraining.

8. Cardiovascular Exercise: Don't neglect cardiovascular exercise like walking, swimming, or cycling, as it complements strength training and promotes overall heart health.

9. Nutrition: Maintain a balanced diet with adequate protein to support muscle growth and repair.

10. Stay Hydrated: Proper hydration is essential for muscle function and overall well-being.

11. Restful Sleep: Ensure you get enough quality sleep to support muscle recovery and overall health.

12. Safety First: Ensure your exercise space is well-lit, free from hazards, and equipped with sturdy handrails if needed.

Sample Strength Training Exercises

Here are some sample exercises to include in your strength training routine:

- Squats: Target your legs and glutes.
- Push-ups: Strengthen your chest, shoulders, and triceps.
- Dumbbell Rows: Work on your upper back and biceps.
- Planks: Engage your core, back, and shoulders.
- Lunges: Focus on your legs and glutes.
- Dumbbell Chest Press: Strengthen your chest and triceps.
- Bicep Curls: Work on your biceps.

Remember that everyone's starting point and progress will be different, so tailor your strength training routine to your abilities and goals. Incremental progress is the key to success.

Boosting muscular strength is not only possible for women over 60 but highly beneficial. It contributes to functional independence, fall prevention, improved bone health, and overall well-being. By incorporating proper resistance training, maintaining a balanced lifestyle, and following safety guidelines, women in this age group can build and maintain muscular strength, leading to a healthier, more vibrant life. Prioritize your health, stay consistent, and enjoy the benefits of a stronger, more resilient body as you age gracefully.

Improving Balance and Stability

Balance and stability are essential aspects of daily life, and they become increasingly crucial as women age, especially those over 60. Good balance and stability reduce the risk of falls and injuries, enhance mobility, and contribute to overall well-being. In this guide, we'll explore the importance of improving balance and stability, the benefits it offers, and practical ways for women over 60 to achieve and maintain them.

The Significance of Balance and Stability

Balance refers to your ability to maintain an upright position and control your body's position while standing, sitting, or moving. Stability is closely related, referring to the body's ability to maintain a steady and controlled posture or position during various activities. Both are integral to everyday life, and here's why they matter for women over 60:

1. Fall Prevention: Balance and stability training can significantly reduce the risk of falls, which become more common as we age. Falls can result in serious injuries, fractures, and a loss of independence.

2. Functional Independence: Good balance and stability are essential for performing daily activities, such as walking, getting up from a chair, or reaching for items on high shelves, without assistance.

3. Enhanced Mobility: Improved balance and stability allow for greater ease of movement and increased flexibility, making it easier to engage in physical activities and hobbies.

4. Reduced Joint Strain: Better stability can help alleviate strain on joints, reducing the risk of joint pain and discomfort.

5. Confidence and Mental Well-being: Feeling stable and balanced enhances confidence and promotes a positive outlook on life.

Benefits of Improving Balance and Stability

For women over 60, there are several compelling benefits associated with enhancing balance and stability:

1. Fall Risk Reduction: Improved balance and stability significantly reduce the risk of falls and related injuries.

2. Enhanced Mobility: Better stability translates into greater mobility and ease of movement, allowing you to enjoy an active lifestyle.

3. Better Posture: Improved balance leads to better posture, reducing the risk of musculoskeletal issues and back pain.

4. Increased Confidence: As your balance and stability improve, you'll feel more confident in various situations, both physically and mentally.

5. Cognitive Benefits: Some research suggests that balance training may have cognitive benefits, helping to sharpen your mind.

Practical Ways to Improve Balance and Stability

Here are some practical strategies and exercises for women over 60 to enhance their balance and stability:

1. Consult a Professional: Before starting any new exercise program, consult with a healthcare provider or physical therapist, especially if you have pre-existing medical conditions or concerns.

2. Balance Training: Incorporate balance exercises into your routine. These can include simple activities like standing on one foot or walking heel-to-toe. Gradually progress to more challenging exercises as you improve.

3. Yoga and Tai Chi: Consider taking up yoga or tai chi classes. These practices combine balance, flexibility, and mental focus and are well-suited for older adults.

4. Strength Training: Building strength in your legs, core, and back can enhance stability. Focus on resistance exercises for these muscle groups.

5. Core Strengthening: A strong core is crucial for stability. Incorporate exercises like planks, bridges, and leg lifts into your routine.

6. Ankle Strengthening: Strong ankles are key to balance. Simple ankle circles and calf raises can help strengthen these areas.

7. Sensory Awareness: Pay attention to sensory cues. Practice exercises with your eyes closed to rely more on proprioception (the body's sense of its position) and less on vision.

8. Supportive Footwear: Ensure you wear comfortable and supportive shoes that provide good grip and stability.

9. Functional Activities: Engage in activities that challenge your balance in a functional way, such as gardening, dancing, or taking leisurely walks on uneven terrain.

10. Balance Tools: Consider using tools like balance boards, stability balls, or foam pads to add variety to your balance training.

11. Progressive Training: Gradually increase the intensity and duration of your balance exercises as you become more confident and stable.

Sample Balance Exercises

Here are some sample balance exercises suitable for women over 60:

1. Single-Leg Stand: Stand on one foot for 30 seconds, gradually increasing the time.

2. Heel-to-Toe Walk: Walk in a straight line with one foot placed directly in front of the other.

3. Leg Swings: Stand near a support and swing one leg forward and backward, then side to side.

4. Standing Clock Reach: Stand on one foot and reach your opposite hand in different directions as if pointing to the hours on a clock.

5. Tai Chi Movements: Practice tai chi movements, which emphasize flowing motions and balance.

6. Yoga Poses: Incorporate yoga poses like tree pose, warrior pose, and chair pose, which challenge balance and flexibility.

Remember that improving balance and stability is a gradual process. It's essential to start at your current level of ability and progress safely. Balance exercises should be done in a controlled environment with proper support if needed. Always prioritize safety and listen to your body's cues.

Improving balance and stability is a valuable investment in your overall well-being, especially for women over 60. By incorporating balance and stability exercises into your routine, seeking professional guidance when necessary, and maintaining a balanced lifestyle, you can enjoy the physical and mental benefits that come with enhanced stability. Embrace the journey towards better balance, and savor the confidence, mobility, and independence it brings to your life as you age gracefully.

Chapter 6

Low-Impact Wall Pilates Workouts

Wall Pilates is an excellent low-impact exercise option for women over 60. It provides the benefits of Pilates while using a wall for support, making it gentle on the joints and accessible for various fitness levels. These low-impact Wall Pilates workouts are designed to improve strength, flexibility, and balance while minimizing the risk of strain or injury.

Warm-Up (5 minutes)
1. Wall Roll-Downs:
    - Stand facing the wall with your feet hip-width apart.
    - Place your hands on the wall at shoulder height.
    - Slowly roll your spine down, vertebra by vertebra, as far as comfortable.
    - Roll back up, stacking your spine one vertebra at a time.
    - Repeat 5 times.

2. Wall Shoulder Rolls:
    - Stand with your back against the wall.
    - Roll your shoulders forward in a circular motion for 30 seconds.
    - Then, roll them backward for another 30 seconds.

Wall Pilates Routine (15 minutes)

3. Wall Squats:
    - Stand facing the wall with your feet hip-width apart.
    - Place your hands on the wall at shoulder height.
    - Lower your body into a squat position, keeping your knees aligned with your ankles.
    - Push through your heels to return to the starting position.
    - Perform 10-12 squats.

4. Wall Leg Lifts:
    - Stand facing the wall, placing your hands on it for support.
    - Lift one leg straight out to the side, keeping it straight.
    - Lower it back down.
    - Perform 10-12 lifts on each leg.

5. Wall Push-Ups:
   - Stand facing the wall with your arms extended at shoulder height, hands on the wall.
   - Step back, keeping your body in a diagonal line, and engage your core.
   - Bend your elbows and lower your chest toward the wall.
   - Push back to the starting position.
   - Perform 10-12 push-ups.

6. Wall Planks:
   - Stand facing the wall and place your hands on it at shoulder height.
   - Step back, extending your body into a plank position.
   - Engage your core and hold the plank for 20-30 seconds.
   - Gradually increase the duration as you become stronger.

Cool Down and Stretching (5 minutes)

7. Wall Calf Stretch:
   - Stand facing the wall with one foot back.
   - Bend your front knee and keep your back leg straight.
   - Lean forward, feeling a stretch in your calf.
   - Hold for 15-20 seconds on each leg.

8. Wall Chest Opener:
    - Stand with your back to the wall.
    - Extend your arms straight back and place your hands against the wall at shoulder height.
    - Gently press your chest forward and upward, feeling a stretch in your chest and shoulders.
    - Hold for 15-20 seconds.

9. Wall Hamstring Stretch:
    - Sit on the floor with your legs extended straight in front of you.
    - Extend one leg up the wall.
    - Reach for your toes, feeling a stretch in your hamstrings.
    - Hold for 15-20 seconds on each leg.

10. Wall Spinal Twist:
    - Sit on a chair with your feet flat on the floor.
    - Cross one leg over the other and gently twist your upper body to the side.
    - Place one hand on the outside of your knee and the other hand on the chair's backrest.
    - Hold for 15-20 seconds on each side.

These low-impact Wall Pilates workouts for women over 60 provide a safe and effective way to improve strength, flexibility, and balance. Always perform exercises with proper form, and listen to your body's cues. If you have any underlying health conditions or concerns, consult with a healthcare professional before starting a new exercise program.

Full-Body Workouts

A full-body workout is an excellent way for women over 60 to maintain overall health and fitness. This routine combines strength, flexibility, and cardiovascular exercises to help you stay active and feel your best. Remember to warm up before starting and cool down at the end of your workout. Always consult with a healthcare provider before beginning a new exercise program, especially if you have any medical conditions or concerns.

Warm-Up (5-10 minutes)

1. March in Place: Start by marching in place to raise your heart rate and warm up your muscles. Swing your arms gently as you march for 2-3 minutes.

2. Arm Circles: Stand with your feet hip-width apart and extend your arms to the sides. Make small circles with your arms, gradually increasing the size

of the circles. After 30 seconds, reverse the direction.

3.Leg Swings: Hold onto a sturdy surface for support. Swing one leg forward and backward, then switch to the other leg. Do this for 1 minute on each leg.

Full-Body Workout Routine (20-30 minutes)

4. Squats:
   - Stand with your feet shoulder-width apart.
   - Lower your body as if you were sitting in a chair, keeping your knees over your ankles.
   - Push through your heels to return to the starting position.
   - Perform 2 sets of 10-12 squats.

5. Wall Push-Ups:
   - Stand facing a wall with your arms extended at shoulder height.
   - Step back and keep your body in a diagonal line.
   - Bend your elbows to lower your chest toward the wall, then push back.
   - Perform 2 sets of 10-12 wall push-ups.

6. Standing Leg Raises:
   - Stand next to a sturdy chair for support.

- Lift one leg out to the side while keeping it straight.
- Lower it back down.
- Perform 2 sets of 10-12 leg raises on each leg.

7. Wall Plank:
   - Stand facing the wall and place your hands on it at shoulder height.
   - Step back and extend your body into a plank position.
   - Engage your core and hold for 20-30 seconds.
   - Gradually increase the duration as you become stronger.

8. Dumbbell Bicep Curls:
   - Hold a light dumbbell in each hand with your arms extended by your sides.
   - Bend your elbows to curl the weights towards your shoulders, then lower them back down.
   - Perform 2 sets of 10-12 curls.

9. Dumbbell Shoulder Press:
   - Hold a dumbbell in each hand at shoulder height.
   - Press the weights overhead, then lower them back down.

- Perform 2 sets of 10-12 shoulder presses.

10. Seated Leg Extensions:
    - Sit on a sturdy chair with your feet flat on the floor.
    - Extend one leg straight out, then lower it back down.
    - Perform 2 sets of 10-12 leg extensions on each leg.

Cool Down and Stretching (5-10 minutes)

11. Deep Breathing: Take a few minutes to perform deep breathing exercises to lower your heart rate and relax your body.

12. Neck and Shoulder Stretch: Gently tilt your head from side to side and perform shoulder rolls to release tension.

13. Standing Quad Stretch: Stand and hold onto a sturdy surface for support. Bend one knee and bring your heel towards your buttocks, holding onto your ankle. Hold for 15-20 seconds on each leg.

14. Standing Calf Stretch: Stand facing a wall with one foot back. Bend your front knee while keeping your back leg straight. Lean forward, feeling a

stretch in your calf. Hold for 15-20 seconds on each leg.

15. Seated Hamstring Stretch: Sit on the floor with your legs extended in front of you. Reach for your toes, feeling a stretch in your hamstrings. Hold for 15-20 seconds.

This full-body workout routine for women over 60 incorporates strength, flexibility, and balance exercises to help you maintain overall fitness and well-being. Perform this routine 2-3 times a week, and remember to listen to your body and modify exercises as needed to match your fitness level and comfort. Stay consistent, and enjoy the benefits of staying active as you age gracefully.

Focused Exercises for Different Needs

As women age, specific exercise needs may arise due to changes in health, fitness goals, and lifestyle. Here are focused exercises tailored to address different needs for women over 60. Consult with a healthcare provider before starting any new exercise program, especially if you have medical conditions or concerns.

For Cardiovascular Health:

1. Brisk Walking: Aim for at least 30 minutes of brisk walking most days of the week to improve heart health, increase stamina, and support weight management.

2. Cycling: Riding a stationary or regular bicycle is a low-impact way to boost cardiovascular fitness. Start with shorter sessions and gradually increase duration.

3. Swimming: Swimming provides a full-body workout with minimal impact on joints. It's excellent for cardiovascular health and overall muscle tone.

For Strength and Muscle Tone:

4. Resistance Training: Incorporate resistance bands, light dumbbells, or bodyweight exercises like squats, lunges, and push-ups to maintain or build muscle strength.

5. Yoga: Regular yoga practice improves flexibility, balance, and muscle tone. Choose yoga classes or routines tailored to your fitness level.

6. Tai Chi: Tai Chi enhances muscular strength, balance, and coordination. It's a gentle yet effective form of exercise for older adults.

For Balance and Stability:

7. Balance Exercises: Include activities like standing on one leg, walking heel-to-toe, or using balance boards to improve stability and reduce the risk of falls.

8. Pilates: Pilates focuses on core strength and stability. Look for classes or routines designed for seniors or beginners.

9. Chair Yoga: Chair yoga adapts traditional yoga poses for seated or supported positions, making it an excellent choice for enhancing balance and flexibility.

For Flexibility:

10. Stretching Routines: Perform daily stretching exercises to maintain or improve flexibility in major muscle groups. Focus on areas prone to stiffness, such as hips, shoulders, and hamstrings.

11. Foam Rolling: Using a foam roller can help release muscle tension and improve flexibility. Gently roll over tight or sore areas for relief.

For Bone Health:

12. Weight-Bearing Exercises: Engage in weight-bearing activities like walking, dancing, or stair climbing to support bone density.

13. Resistance Bands: Use resistance bands for exercises that target the major muscle groups, which can help maintain bone strength.

For Stress Reduction and Mental Well-being:

14. Mindfulness Meditation: Practice mindfulness meditation to reduce stress, improve focus, and enhance overall mental well-being.

15. Deep Breathing Exercises: Incorporate deep breathing exercises throughout the day to manage stress and promote relaxation.

For Joint Health:

16. Low-Impact Aerobics: Engage in low-impact aerobic workouts like water aerobics to protect your joints while staying active.

17. Range of Motion Exercises: Perform gentle range of motion exercises to keep joints mobile and reduce stiffness.

For Weight Management:

18. Calorie-Burning Activities: Choose activities that help you burn calories, such as dancing, hiking, or playing recreational sports.

19. Portion Control: Combine exercise with a balanced diet and mindful portion control to manage weight effectively.

Remember that consistency is key to reaping the benefits of exercise. It's essential to tailor your exercise routine to your specific needs and gradually progress as you become more comfortable with each activity. Stay hydrated, get adequate rest, and prioritize safety while exercising. Listen to your body, and don't hesitate to modify exercises or seek professional guidance when needed. With the right approach, regular physical activity can enhance your health and well-being throughout your life.

8. Progression and Challenges
Progression and Challenges for Wall Pilates for Women Over 60

Wall Pilates is an excellent low-impact exercise option for women over 60, but it's important to progressively challenge yourself while being mindful of potential limitations and challenges. Here's how to progress your Wall Pilates practice and address common challenges:

Progression:

1. Start Slowly: If you're new to Wall Pilates, begin with the basics. Perform foundational exercises to build strength, flexibility, and balance before progressing to more advanced movements.

2. Increase Repetitions: As you become more comfortable with an exercise, gradually increase the number of repetitions. For example, if you started with 10 repetitions, work towards 15 or 20.

3. Add Resistance: To increase the challenge, consider using resistance bands or light dumbbells during some exercises. This can enhance muscle engagement and strength-building.

4. Extend Hold Times: For exercises involving static holds, like wall planks, gradually increase the duration. Start with 20-30 seconds and work your way up to 60 seconds or more.

5. Explore Variations: Look for variations of Wall Pilates exercises that target different muscle groups or provide a more significant challenge. For example, you can progress from Wall Squats to One-Legged Wall Squats.

6. Incorporate Advanced Moves: Once you've mastered the fundamentals, explore advanced Wall Pilates movements like Wall Angels, Wall Scissor Legs, or Wall Teasers. These exercises require more core strength and balance.

7. Combine Movements: Create flow sequences by combining multiple Wall Pilates exercises. This adds complexity and engages various muscle groups simultaneously.

Challenges:

1. Balance and Stability: Maintaining balance can be challenging, especially if you have balance issues or are new to Pilates. Use the wall for support when needed and start with simple balance exercises like one-legged stands.

2. Flexibility Limitations: If you have limited flexibility, certain movements may be challenging.

Focus on gentle stretching exercises to improve flexibility over time.

3. Strength Limitations: Building strength takes time. Don't get discouraged if you can't perform advanced exercises immediately. Start with basic strength-building exercises and progress gradually.

4. Safety: Ensure your exercise space is safe, well-lit, and free from obstacles. Use a sturdy chair or wall for support when necessary, especially during balance exercises.

5. Proper Form: Maintaining correct form is crucial to prevent injury and maximize the benefits of Wall Pilates. Consider working with a certified Pilates instructor to ensure proper technique.

6. Overexertion: Avoid overexertion or pushing yourself too hard, especially if you have pre-existing medical conditions. Listen to your body and adjust the intensity as needed.

7. Consultation: Always consult with a healthcare provider before starting a new exercise program, especially if you have underlying health concerns or recent injuries.

8. Modifications: Be prepared to modify exercises to suit your individual needs. Pilates can be adapted to accommodate various fitness levels and physical limitations.

9. Breathing: Proper breathing is integral to Pilates. Focus on coordinating your breath with movement, as it can enhance the effectiveness of exercises.

10. Patience: Progress may be gradual, so be patient with yourself. Celebrate small victories and stay consistent in your practice.

Remember that Wall Pilates should be enjoyable and beneficial to your overall health. With time, dedication, and a mindful approach to progression and addressing challenges, you can experience the positive effects of this gentle yet effective exercise method for women over 60.

Advancing Your Wall Pilates Practice

Advancing your Wall Pilates practice as a woman over 60 can be a rewarding journey towards improved strength, flexibility, and overall well-being. Here are steps and tips to help you progress in your practice while ensuring safety and enjoyment:

1. **Build a Strong Foundation:**

- Start with the basics: Ensure you have a solid understanding of fundamental Wall Pilates exercises and proper form.
- Focus on breath: Master the coordination of breath with movement, which is essential in Pilates.
- Develop core strength: Strengthen your core muscles, as they play a central role in Wall Pilates.

2. **Gradual Progression:**
- Increase repetitions: Gradually add more repetitions to exercises as your strength improves. Start with 10-12 repetitions and work your way up.
- Extend hold times: For static exercises, like wall planks, aim to hold for longer durations, progressively increasing from 20-30 seconds to 60 seconds or more.
- Add resistance: Incorporate resistance bands or light dumbbells to some exercises for added challenge.
- Explore advanced movements: As you become more comfortable, explore

advanced Wall Pilates movements that engage multiple muscle groups simultaneously.

3. **Experiment with Variations**:
   - Target different muscle groups: Explore variations of Wall Pilates exercises that work on specific muscle groups or provide a different challenge.
   - Combine movements: Create flow sequences by combining multiple Wall Pilates exercises to make your practice more dynamic.

4. **Seek Professional Guidance**:
   - Consider working with a certified Pilates instructor: A qualified instructor can provide personalized guidance, correct your form, and introduce advanced exercises safely.
   - Join group classes: Participate in group Wall Pilates classes tailored for women over 60. Group dynamics can be motivating and educational.

5. **Balance and Stability:**
   - Continue working on balance: Balance exercises are crucial, so don't neglect them. You can advance to more challenging balance poses over time.

- Practice proprioception: Develop a sense of your body's position in space by incorporating exercises with your eyes closed.

6. **Flexibility and Stretching**:
    - Regularly incorporate stretching exercises: Maintain or improve flexibility by incorporating gentle stretching routines into your practice.
    - Focus on areas of stiffness: Pay particular attention to areas prone to stiffness, such as hips, shoulders, and hamstrings.

7. **Safety and Modifications**:
    - Listen to your body: Always prioritize safety and listen to your body. If an exercise causes discomfort or pain, modify it or skip it.
    - Use props for support: Don't hesitate to use props like a sturdy chair or the wall for support during exercises.
    - Modify exercises: Be prepared to modify exercises to suit your individual needs and physical limitations.

8. **Stay Consistent**:

- Consistency is key: Regular practice is essential for progress. Aim for at least 2-3 sessions per week to see improvements.
- Patience and persistence: Understand that progress may be gradual, so be patient with yourself and stay persistent in your practice.

Advancing your Wall Pilates practice for women over 60 is a journey that can lead to improved physical and mental well-being. With a gradual and mindful approach, you can continue to enjoy the benefits of this gentle yet effective exercise method while challenging yourself and reaching new levels of strength and flexibility.

Taking It to the Next Level

Taking your fitness to the next level as a woman over 60 can be an empowering and rewarding journey. It's important to do so in a safe and mindful manner to enjoy continued health and well-being. Here are some steps to help you take your fitness to the next level:

1. Set Clear Goals: Define your fitness goals, whether it's improving strength, endurance, flexibility, or achieving specific fitness milestones.

2. Consult a Professional: Consider working with a certified personal trainer or fitness coach who specializes in training for older adults. They can create a customized plan and ensure proper guidance.

3. Progressive Strength Training: Continue strength training with progressively heavier weights or resistance bands. Aim for 2-3 strength training sessions per week, targeting all major muscle groups.

4. Cardiovascular Fitness: Increase the intensity and duration of your cardiovascular workouts. Gradually work your way up to more challenging exercises like high-intensity interval training (HIIT) or advanced aerobics classes.

5. Flexibility and Mobility: Focus on improving flexibility and mobility with regular stretching, yoga, or Pilates sessions. These activities can enhance range of motion and reduce the risk of injuries.

6. Nutrition and Hydration: Pay attention to your diet, ensuring it supports your fitness goals. Adequate hydration and a balanced diet are essential for energy and recovery.

7. Mindfulness and Recovery:
    - Incorporate mindfulness practices like meditation and deep breathing to manage stress and improve mental well-being.
    - Prioritize rest and recovery days to allow your body to heal and grow stronger.

8. Challenge Your Comfort Zone:
    - Try new activities or fitness classes that push your boundaries and keep your workouts engaging.

9. Social Support:
    - Join fitness groups, classes, or workout with friends to stay motivated and accountable.

10. Track Your Progress:
    - Keep a fitness journal to track your workouts, progress, and any changes in your health and fitness levels.

11. Listen to Your Body:
    - Pay close attention to your body's cues. If you experience pain or discomfort, modify exercises or consult a healthcare provider.

12. Celebrate Achievements:

- Celebrate your milestones and achievements along the way. Recognize the progress you've made and stay motivated.

13. Stay Informed:
    - Continually educate yourself on fitness, nutrition, and wellness topics relevant to your age group. Knowledge can empower you to make informed choices.

14. Adapt to Changing Needs:
    - Be flexible and willing to adapt your fitness routine to changing needs and circumstances. It's natural for your body to have different requirements as you age.

15. Enjoy the Journey:
    - Embrace the journey of self-improvement and take pride in your commitment to health and fitness. Enjoy the physical and mental benefits that come with it.

Remember that fitness is a lifelong journey, and there's no age limit to achieving your goals. By taking a mindful and progressive approach, you can continue to challenge yourself, stay active, and maintain a high quality of life as a woman over 60.

Chapter 8

Recovery and Self-Care

Recovery and self-care are essential aspects of maintaining overall health and well-being, especially for women over 60. Prioritizing self-care can help you recover from physical activity, manage stress, and promote a healthy, balanced lifestyle. Here are some recovery and self-care tips tailored for women in this age group:

1. **Prioritize Rest:**
1. Quality Sleep: Ensure you get 7-9 hours of quality sleep each night. Create a calming bedtime routine and maintain a consistent sleep schedule.

2. Rest Days: Incorporate rest days into your exercise routine. These days allow your body to recover and prevent overexertion.

2. **Nutrition and Hydration**:
3. Balanced Diet: Consume a well-balanced diet rich in fruits, vegetables, lean proteins, whole grains, and healthy fats. Pay attention to portion control and avoid excessive processed foods.

4. Stay Hydrated: Drink an adequate amount of water throughout the day to maintain proper bodily functions and support recovery.

5. Post-Workout Nutrition: After exercise, consume a combination of protein and carbohydrates to aid muscle recovery and replenish energy stores.

3. **Stretching and Mobility**:
6. Stretch Regularly: Incorporate daily stretching routines to improve flexibility and reduce the risk of injury. Focus on areas prone to tightness.

7. Yoga or Pilates: Consider participating in yoga or Pilates classes, which can enhance flexibility, balance, and relaxation.

4. **Stress Management**:
8. Meditation and Deep Breathing: Practice mindfulness meditation and deep breathing exercises to reduce stress and promote relaxation.

9. Hobbies and Leisure Activities: Engage in hobbies and activities you enjoy to unwind and take your mind off daily stressors.

5. **Self-Care Practices**:

10. Massage Therapy: Consider occasional massages to release muscle tension and promote relaxation.

11. Hot Baths: Soaking in a warm bath with Epsom salts can soothe sore muscles and provide relaxation.

12. Self-Massage: Use foam rollers or massage balls to perform self-myofascial release to relieve muscle tightness.

6. **Regular Check-ups**:

13. Health Screenings: Schedule regular check-ups and health screenings to monitor your overall health and address any medical concerns promptly.

14. Consult Specialists: If you have specific health conditions or concerns, consult specialists, such as a physical therapist, nutritionist, or mental health professional, to address your unique needs.

7. **Social Connection**:

15. Stay Connected: Maintain social connections with friends and family. Socializing can improve mental well-being.

16. Support Groups: Consider joining support groups or communities tailored to your interests or health conditions to connect with like-minded individuals.

8. Mind-Body Connection:

17. Positive Self-Talk: Practice positive self-talk and self-compassion. Encourage yourself with affirmations and focus on self-acceptance.

18. Mindfulness Practices: Engage in mindfulness practices, such as mindful eating or mindful walking, to connect with your body and emotions.

9. Adapt to Individual Needs:

19. Listen to Your Body: Pay attention to your body's signals and adapt your self-care routine as needed. Modify activities or seek professional guidance when necessary.

10. Enjoy Life:

20. Pursue Joy: Prioritize activities and experiences that bring you joy and fulfillment. Embrace life's pleasures and cherish meaningful moments.

Remember that self-care is not a luxury but a necessity for maintaining health and vitality as a woman over 60. By incorporating these practices into your daily life, you can promote physical and mental well-being, enhance recovery, and enjoy a fulfilling and balanced lifestyle.

Restorative Practices

Restorative practices are essential for promoting relaxation, reducing stress, and enhancing overall well-being, particularly for women over 60. These practices prioritize rest and rejuvenation to support physical, mental, and emotional health. Here are some restorative practices tailored for this age group:

1. Meditation:
Meditation is a powerful tool for calming the mind, reducing stress, and enhancing mental clarity. Consider incorporating meditation into your daily routine. You can start with short sessions and gradually extend the duration. Guided meditation apps or classes designed for seniors can be helpful.

2. Deep Breathing Exercises:
Deep breathing exercises promote relaxation and reduce anxiety. Practice deep breathing techniques regularly, especially during stressful moments.

Simple exercises like diaphragmatic breathing or the 4-7-8 technique can be effective.

3. Gentle Yoga:
Gentle yoga classes or routines tailored for seniors are ideal for enhancing flexibility, balance, and relaxation. Yoga poses, combined with controlled breathing, can help alleviate tension and promote a sense of calm.

4. Tai Chi:
Tai Chi is a low-impact martial art that focuses on slow, flowing movements. It enhances balance, coordination, and mindfulness. Look for Tai Chi classes specifically designed for older adults.

5. Progressive Muscle Relaxation:
Progressive muscle relaxation involves tensing and releasing different muscle groups to promote relaxation. It's an effective way to relieve physical tension and stress.

6. Warm Baths:
Taking warm baths with Epsom salts can relax your muscles, ease joint discomfort, and provide a sense of relaxation. Consider adding aromatherapy oils like lavender for added relaxation.

7. Restorative Yoga:

Restorative yoga is a practice that involves holding gentle poses with the support of props like blankets and bolsters. It encourages deep relaxation and stress relief.

8. Mindful Walking:
Take mindful walks in nature to connect with the environment and clear your mind. Focus on your surroundings, your breathing, and the sensations in your body.

9. Journaling:
Keeping a journal allows you to express your thoughts and emotions, providing a sense of release and clarity. You can write about your experiences, gratitude, or daily reflections.

10. Creative Activities:
Engage in creative activities such as painting, drawing, knitting, or crafting. These activities can be therapeutic and provide a sense of accomplishment.

11. Reading and Listening:
Enjoy reading books, listening to soothing music, or engaging in audiobooks that inspire relaxation. Select materials that uplift your mood and encourage tranquility.

12. Nature Connection:
Spend time outdoors and connect with nature. Whether it's gardening, bird-watching, or simply sitting in a peaceful garden, nature can have a calming effect.

13. Social Connection:
Maintain social connections with friends and family. Spending quality time with loved ones can provide emotional support and promote relaxation.

14. Restorative Sleep:
Prioritize sleep by establishing a consistent bedtime routine and creating a comfortable sleep environment. Adequate sleep is essential for overall well-being.

Remember that restorative practices should be incorporated into your daily or weekly routine to reap their full benefits. They provide opportunities for relaxation, self-care, and inner peace, helping you navigate life's challenges with greater resilience and a sense of calm.

Self-Care Tips for Women Over 60

Self-care is vital for women over 60 to maintain physical, mental, and emotional well-being. Here are some self-care tips tailored for this age group:

1. Prioritize Sleep: Ensure you get enough quality sleep each night. Create a comfortable sleep environment, maintain a consistent sleep schedule, and practice relaxation techniques before bedtime.

2. Stay Physically Active: Engage in regular physical activity that suits your fitness level and preferences. Activities like walking, swimming, yoga, or tai chi can help improve strength, flexibility, and overall health.

3. Healthy Eating: Maintain a balanced diet rich in fruits, vegetables, lean proteins, whole grains, and healthy fats. Pay attention to portion control and stay hydrated.

4. Regular Health Check-ups: Schedule regular check-ups and health screenings to monitor your overall health and address any medical concerns promptly.

5. Mindfulness and Relaxation: Practice mindfulness meditation, deep breathing exercises, or yoga to reduce stress and promote relaxation.

6. Social Connections: Stay connected with friends and family. Socializing and maintaining meaningful relationships contribute to emotional well-being.

7. Hobbies and Interests: Pursue hobbies and interests that bring you joy and fulfillment. It can be painting, gardening, reading, or anything that ignites your passion.

8. Stay Informed: Continually educate yourself on topics of interest or new skills. Learning can be a fulfilling and enriching self-care practice.

9. Positive Self-Talk: Replace self-criticism with self-compassion and positive self-talk. Embrace your unique qualities and value.

10. Relaxation Techniques: Explore relaxation techniques such as taking warm baths, practicing progressive muscle relaxation, or enjoying nature.

11. Limit Stressors: Identify and manage sources of stress in your life. Simplify your daily routines and prioritize tasks to reduce unnecessary stress.

12. Seek Professional Help: Don't hesitate to consult professionals, such as therapists or counselors, for mental health support if needed. Your emotional well-being is crucial.

13. Stay Hydrated: Drink an adequate amount of water throughout the day to support overall health and vitality.

14. Balance Activities: Find a balance between activities and rest. It's important to avoid overextending yourself and allow time for relaxation.

15. Stay Active Mentally: Keep your mind active by engaging in puzzles, brain games, or learning new skills. Mental stimulation is important for cognitive health.

16. Stay Organized: Organize your living space and create routines that enhance efficiency and reduce daily stressors.

17. Gentle Self-Care Practices: Engage in gentle self-care practices such as massages, spa days, or simply treating yourself to small indulgences.

18. Laugh and Enjoy Life: Embrace humor and laughter as part of your daily life. Enjoying

light-hearted moments can boost your mood and reduce stress.

19. Express Gratitude: Practice gratitude by acknowledging the positive aspects of your life. It can be helpful to keep a gratitude journal.

20. Adapt to Changing Needs: Recognize that self-care needs may change over time. Be flexible and willing to adapt your self-care routine to your current circumstances.

Remember that self-care is not selfish; it's essential for your health and well-being. By making self-care a priority in your life, you can enhance your quality of life and navigate the aging process with grace and vitality.

Building Consistency

Consistency is key to maintaining a healthy and active lifestyle for women over 60. Here are some strategies to help you build and maintain consistency in your daily routines and activities:

1. Set Clear Goals: Define your health and wellness goals. Having clear objectives will motivate you to stay consistent in working towards them.

2. Create a Routine: Establish a daily or weekly routine that incorporates exercise, self-care, and healthy habits. Having a structured schedule can help you stay on track.

3. Start Small: Begin with manageable goals and activities. Gradually increase the duration and intensity as you become more comfortable and confident.

4. Use a Planner: Use a planner or digital calendar to schedule your workouts, meal planning, and self-care activities. Seeing your commitments can help you stay accountable.

5. Accountability Partner: Partner with a friend or family member who shares your goals. Having someone to exercise with or check in on your progress can boost motivation.

6. Track Your Progress: Keep a journal to record your activities, workouts, and achievements. Tracking progress can be rewarding and motivating.

7. Variety in Activities: Mix up your workouts and activities to prevent boredom. Try different exercises, classes, or hobbies to keep things interesting.

8. Prioritize Self-Care: Recognize the importance of self-care. Make time for relaxation, meditation, and activities that bring you joy and reduce stress.

9. Prepare Ahead: Plan your meals and snacks in advance to ensure you make healthy choices throughout the day. Meal prepping can simplify your nutrition routine.

10. Rest and Recovery: Include rest days in your fitness routine to allow your body to recover. Overexertion can lead to burnout and inconsistency.

11. Adapt to Life Changes: Be flexible and willing to adapt your routine when life circumstances change. Modify your plan rather than giving up entirely.

12. Positive Self-Talk: Practice positive self-talk and self-compassion. Encourage yourself and focus on your accomplishments, no matter how small they may seem.

13. Stay Informed: Continually educate yourself about health and wellness topics relevant to your age group. Knowledge can empower you to make informed choices.

14. Mindful Adjustments: Listen to your body and make mindful adjustments as needed. If an activity causes discomfort, consider modifying it or seeking professional guidance.

15. Celebrate Achievements: Celebrate your milestones and achievements along the way. Small victories deserve recognition.

16. Stay Motivated: Revisit your goals regularly and remind yourself of why you started. Stay connected to your motivations to maintain consistency.

17. Incorporate Fun: Engage in activities that you genuinely enjoy. Fun and enjoyment can be powerful motivators.

Remember that consistency is a gradual process. It's okay to have occasional setbacks or deviations from your routine. The key is to stay committed to your long-term health and well-being. By implementing these strategies, you can build and maintain consistency in your daily habits and routines, leading to a happier and healthier life as a woman over 60.

Conclusion

Achieving Your Wellness Goals

As a woman over 60, achieving your wellness goals is an empowering journey that can greatly enhance your quality of life. Throughout this process, you've learned the importance of setting clear objectives, creating a structured routine, and staying consistent in your efforts. You've discovered the value of self-care, positive self-talk, and flexibility in adapting to life's changes.

Remember that achieving wellness goals is not a one-time accomplishment but an ongoing commitment to your health and well-being. It's about making small, sustainable changes that lead to long-lasting improvements in your physical, mental, and emotional health.

In this journey, you've also recognized the significance of balance—balancing your physical activity with rest, balancing your nutrition with occasional indulgence, and balancing your goals with self-compassion. Wellness is about harmony, not perfection.

Celebrate your achievements, both big and small, and continue to set new goals to keep your journey exciting and motivating. Surround yourself with a supportive community, whether it's friends, family, or like-minded individuals who share your wellness aspirations.

Ultimately, your wellness goals are a testament to your commitment to living a vibrant, fulfilling life. Embrace this journey with an open heart, an adventurous spirit, and the knowledge that you have the power to shape your own well-being for years to come. Your wellness journey is an ongoing story, and the pen is in your hand. Write it with vitality, purpose, and joy.

As you embark on the journey of achieving your wellness goals as a woman over 60, it's important to recognize the profound impact it can have on your life. Through dedication, perseverance, and a commitment to self-care, you have the power to transform your well-being and embrace a vibrant and fulfilling future.

Your wellness goals reflect your unwavering commitment to self-improvement and self-care. They are a testament to your resilience, inner strength, and the wisdom that comes with age. As you've navigated this path, you've discovered that achieving wellness is not a destination but a lifelong expedition.

In the process, you've set clear intentions and established a structured routine that accommodates your unique needs and preferences. You've learned the art of consistency, recognizing that it's the small, deliberate actions taken each day that yield the most significant results over time.

Your wellness journey has also taught you the value of self-compassion. You've discovered that it's perfectly acceptable to have setbacks and moments of indulgence. These are not failures but opportunities to learn, grow, and recalibrate your path towards health and happiness.

Throughout your journey, you've harnessed the power of a positive mindset and self-affirmation. You've embraced the idea that wellness is not just about physical health but also mental and emotional well-being. You've practiced mindfulness, deep breathing, and relaxation techniques to find balance amidst life's demands.

In achieving your wellness goals, you've celebrated each achievement, both big and small. These celebrations are not merely milestones; they are reminders of your resilience and your ability to overcome obstacles. They are a testament to your unwavering commitment to self-improvement.

As you continue this journey, remember that wellness is not a fixed destination but a dynamic state that evolves with time. Embrace change, adapt to new challenges, and remain open to exploration. Your wellness goals are an invitation to embrace the richness of life, to savor its joys, and to confront its complexities with grace and courage.

Surround yourself with a supportive community of friends, family, and kindred spirits who share your aspirations. Share your experiences, offer encouragement, and draw inspiration from those around you.

Your wellness goals are a reflection of your enduring vitality and your commitment to living life to the fullest. They are a testament to the fact that age is not a limitation but an opportunity for growth and renewal. Continue to write your wellness story with purpose, passion, and an unwavering belief in the power of self-care and self-improvement. The canvas of your well-being is vast, and every brushstroke is an affirmation of your remarkable journey towards a healthier, happier, and more vibrant you.

Embracing a Healthier Lifestyle

Embracing a healthier lifestyle as a woman over 60 is not merely a choice; it's a profound declaration of self-love and self-care. It's a journey that encompasses your physical, mental, and emotional well-being, and it holds the promise of a more fulfilling and vibrant life.

Throughout this transformative journey, you've learned to prioritize physical activity, realizing that movement is the foundation of vitality. You've discovered the joy in staying active, whether through brisk walks in nature, gentle yoga sessions, or engaging in activities that invigorate your spirit.

Nutrition has become a source of nourishment and empowerment. You've embraced a balanced diet that fuels your body with essential nutrients, paying heed to portion control and mindful eating. You've come to understand that the food you consume is not only sustenance but also a powerful tool for healing and longevity.

Mindfulness has woven itself into your daily life. You've discovered the art of savoring each moment, practicing gratitude, and finding serenity in the present. Mindful practices have allowed you to make conscious choices that support your well-being and bring harmony to your existence.

Your commitment to a healthier lifestyle is a testament to your resilience and your unwavering belief in the possibilities of self-improvement, regardless of age. You've recognized that age is not a limitation but a canvas upon which you can paint a vibrant, purposeful, and fulfilling life.

In your journey, you've found balance, both in the physical activities that nurture your body and the self-care practices that nourish your soul. You've become attuned to the importance of rest and recovery, understanding that rejuvenation is an integral part of a healthier lifestyle.

Your circle of well-being has expanded to include a supportive community of friends, family, and like-minded individuals. Sharing your experiences, offering encouragement, and drawing inspiration from one another have made the journey richer and more rewarding.

As you conclude this reflection on embracing a healthier lifestyle, remember that this is not a journey with an end point but a lifelong commitment. Continue to seek new adventures, to explore uncharted territories, and to embrace change with grace and enthusiasm.

Celebrate your achievements, for they are not just milestones but reminders of your strength and determination. Each step you've taken towards a healthier lifestyle is a testament to your enduring vitality and your capacity for renewal.

Embrace your healthier lifestyle with an open heart, a curious spirit, and an unwavering belief in your ability to craft a future filled with well-being and fulfillment. Your journey is a testament to the enduring power of self-love and self-care, and it continues to unfold with the promise of a brighter, healthier, and more vibrant tomorrow.

Bouns

30-Day Wall Pilates Workouts Challenge for Women Over 60

Welcome to the 30-Day Wall Pilates Workouts Challenge designed specifically for women over 60. This challenge will help you enhance your strength, flexibility, and balance using the support of a wall. Each day, you'll focus on different Pilates exercises that gradually progress in intensity. Remember to consult with a healthcare professional before starting any new exercise routine, especially if you have underlying health conditions. Let's get started!

Day 1 - Wall Squats
- Stand with your back against the wall and feet hip-width apart.
- Slide down the wall into a squat position, knees at a 90-degree angle.
- Hold for 20 seconds and repeat 3 times.

Day 2 - Wall Angels**
- Stand with your back against the wall, arms at your sides.
- Slowly raise your arms overhead, keeping them in contact with the wall.

- Lower your arms back to your sides. Repeat for 3 sets of 10.

Day 3 - Wall Planks
- Face the wall, place your hands on it shoulder-width apart.
- Step back, keeping your body in a straight line.
- Hold the plank position for 20 seconds, repeat 3 times.

Day 4 - Wall Bridge
- Lie on your back with your feet flat against the wall and knees bent.
- Lift your hips off the ground, forming a straight line from shoulders to knees.
- Hold for 15 seconds, repeat 3 times.

Day 5 - Wall Leg Lifts
- Lie on your back with your legs extended up the wall.
- Lift one leg up towards the ceiling while keeping the other against the wall.
- Lower and switch legs. Do 3 sets of 10 for each leg.

Day 6 - Wall Push-Ups
- Stand facing the wall with your arms extended at shoulder height.

- Lean in and perform push-ups against the wall. Do 3 sets of 10.

Day 7 - Wall Sit
- Sit against the wall with your knees bent at a 90-degree angle.
- Hold for 30 seconds, repeat 3 times.

Day 8 - Wall Abdominal Curl
- Lie on your back with your feet against the wall and knees bent.
- Curl your upper body off the ground, engaging your core.
- Repeat for 3 sets of 12.

Day 9 - Wall Stretching Routine
- Spend 15 minutes doing various stretches against the wall to improve flexibility.

Day 10 - Wall Side Leg Raises
- Lie on your side with your legs extended up the wall.
- Lift your top leg as high as comfortable, then lower it. Do 3 sets of 10 for each leg.

Day 11 - Wall Bird-Dog
- Stand facing the wall and extend one arm forward and the opposite leg back.
- Repeat for 3 sets of 10 for each side.

Day 12 - Wall Plank with Leg Lift
- Perform a wall plank as on Day 3 but lift one leg at a time. Hold each leg lift for 10 seconds. Do 3 sets.

Day 13 - Wall Scissor Kicks
- Lie on your back with your hips close to the wall and your legs extended up it.
- Cross your right leg over your left and then switch.
- Do 3 sets of 15 scissor kicks for each leg.

Day 14 - Wall Plank Leg Circles
- Perform a wall plank as on Day 3.
- Lift one leg and make small circles in one direction, then reverse. Do 3 sets of 10 circles for each leg.

Day 15 - Wall Pilates Push-Ups
- Stand facing the wall and place your hands on it shoulder-width apart.
- Perform push-ups, keeping your body straight. Do 3 sets of 12.

Day 16 - Wall Pilates Saw
- Sit on the floor with your legs extended wide.

- Reach your right hand towards your left foot, twist your torso.
- Repeat on the other side. Do 3 sets of 10 on each side.

Day 17 - Wall Hip Flexor Stretch
- Stand a few feet from the wall and place your right foot against it.
- Lean forward, feeling the stretch in your hip flexor.
- Hold for 20 seconds on each side.

Day 18 - Wall Roll-Downs
- Stand with your back against the wall, feet hip-width apart.
- Slowly roll down one vertebra at a time, then roll back up.
- Do 3 sets of 10.

Day 19 - Wall Plank Hip Drops
- Perform a wall plank as on Day 3.
- Dip your hips to the right and then to the left. Do 3 sets of 10 on each side.

Day 20 - Wall Pilates Swimming
- Lie on your stomach facing away from the wall.
- Lift your arms, chest, and legs off the ground, fluttering your arms and legs.

- Do this for 3 sets of 20 seconds.

Day 21 - Wall Pilates Teaser
1. Ok Sit with your back against the wall and legs extended.
2. Roll down to your back and then back up to a seated position.
3. Do 3 sets of 10.

Day 22 - Wall Plank Knee Tucks
- Perform a wall plank as on Day 3.
- Bring your right knee towards your chest, then switch legs.
- Do 3 sets of 15 for each leg.

Day 23 - Wall Child's Pose Stretch
- Kneel facing the wall with your arms extended.
- Lower your chest towards the wall and stretch your arms.
- Hold for 30 seconds.

Day 24 - Wall Pilates Leg Circles
- Lie on your back with your legs extended up the wall.
- Make large circles with one leg, then switch directions. Do 3 sets of 10 circles for each leg.

Day 25 - Wall Pilates Twist
- Stand facing the wall and hold your arms out to the sides.
- Twist your torso to the right and then to the left. Do 3 sets of 15 on each side.

Day 26 - Wall Plank with Arm Lift
- Perform a wall plank as on Day 3.
- Lift your right arm off the wall, then switch to the left arm.
- Do 3 sets of 10 on each side.

Day 27 - Wall Pilates Roll Up
- Sit with your back against the wall, legs extended.
- Roll down one vertebra at a time, then roll back up.
- Do 3 sets of 10.

Day 28 - Wall Calf Stretch
- Stand facing the wall with your hands against it.
- Step your right foot back, keeping it flat on the ground to stretch the calf.
- Hold for 20 seconds on each side.

Day 29 - Wall Pilates Push-Ups with Leg Lift
- Stand facing the wall with your hands on it shoulder-width apart.

- Perform a push-up and lift one leg at the top of each push-up.
- Do 3 sets of 12 with alternating leg lifts.

Day 30 - Wall Plank for Max Time
- Perform a wall plank as on Day 3
- Challenge yourself to hold it for as long as possible, aiming for improvement from your Day 3 time.

Congratulations on completing the 30-Day Wall Pilates Workouts Challenge! By now, you should feel more flexible, stronger, and more balanced. Continue to incorporate these exercises into your regular routine to maintain your progress and enjoy the numerous benefits of Wall Pilates. Remember to always prioritize safety and listen to your body.

Day 25 - Wall Pilates Twist
- Stand facing the wall and hold your arms out to the sides.
- Twist your torso to the right and then to the left. Do 3 sets of 15 on each side.

Day 26 - Wall Plank with Arm Lift
- Perform a wall plank as on Day 3.
- Lift your right arm off the wall, then switch to the left arm.
- Do 3 sets of 10 on each side.

Day 27 - Wall Pilates Roll Up
- Sit with your back against the wall, legs extended.
- Roll down one vertebra at a time, then roll back up.
- Do 3 sets of 10.

Day 28 - Wall Calf Stretch
- Stand facing the wall with your hands against it.
- Step your right foot back, keeping it flat on the ground to stretch the calf.
- Hold for 20 seconds on each side.

Day 29 - Wall Pilates Push-Ups with Leg Lift
- Stand facing the wall with your hands on it shoulder-width apart.

- Perform a push-up and lift one leg at the top of each push-up.
- Do 3 sets of 12 with alternating leg lifts.

Day 30 - Wall Plank for Max Time
- Perform a wall plank as on Day 3
- Challenge yourself to hold it for as long as possible, aiming for improvement from your Day 3 time.

Congratulations on completing the 30-Day Wall Pilates Workouts Challenge! By now, you should feel more flexible, stronger, and more balanced. Continue to incorporate these exercises into your regular routine to maintain your progress and enjoy the numerous benefits of Wall Pilates. Remember to always prioritize safety and listen to your body.

The Sensitively Thin Bill of the Shag

Prizewinning Short Stories and Poetry
from
Biscuit Publishing Competition 2003

Biscuit Publishing Ltd
PO Box 123, Washington
Newcastle-upon-Tyne
NE37 2YW
United Kingdom

Published 2003 by
Biscuit Publishing Ltd
PO Box 123, Washington
Newcastle upon Tyne
NE37 2YW

www.biscuitpublishing.com
e-mail: info@biscuitpublishing.com

ISBN 1-903914-11-6

All rights reserved

Copyright of stories, poems and judges' comments remains with the individual authors © 2003

Typeset by Mike Wilson, Bridlington

Cover design by Peter Lister © 2003

Printed in Great Britain by
Jasprint Ltd, NE37 2SH

Contents

Judges' Comments
  Subhadassi   5
  Denise Robertson   6
  Peter Lister   6

Sue Vickerman
  The Sensitively Thin Bill
    of the Shag   11
  Trelleborg to Sassnitz   11
  Waiting for Puffins   12
  Skylark   13
  Stonehaven Harbour   13

Tracey Fuller
  The System Was Turned On   14

Lee Morris
  Female Study I: On the Scent   19
  Female Study II: Self-portrait   19
  Female Study III: Bernadette   20
  Female Study IV: Babushka   21
  Female Study V: Glass Eye   22

Stephen Wade
  Get Lost   23

Doreen Hinchliffe
  In Café Picasso   29
  Intermezzo   29
  Trick of Fortune   30
  Happy Ever After   31
  Things Are Never What
    They Seem   32

Peter Bromley
  Archaeology   33

Andrew Neil Blewitt
  The Epistles to the Brassicans   38
  Harriss   39
  Never Time to Say Goodbye   40
  My Sainted Aunt   41
  The Elder Son Speaks Out   42

Sue Vickerman
  Trekkie   43

Sylvia Goodman
  Skilled Worker   50
  Plea   50
  Fragile Memories   51
  African Statue   52
  Bad Weather Coming   53

Sean Burn
  hard walkin yr old mans
    shadow   54

David Swann
  Boggarts   57
  Pleasure   58
  Ghost Train   59
  The Angel of Old Men's Shins   59
  In the Grotto   60

Noreen Rees
  Jesus on a Nan Bread   62

Jacqui Rowe
  Before the Funeral   67
  Unexposed   68
  Poisoning the Garden   68
  She Means Distant Lies   69
  Seeing Puppies in the Dark   70

Jay Merill
  Timeshare   73

John Halladay
  Hartwig, Hermann and
    Hartmut   78
  The Second Day that Jude
    Calls It the First Day   78
  Mementoes of a Great
    Adventurer   79
  A North Cove Evening   80
  Any Pulp's Sufficient, Mulched
    with Sugar by a Cretin   80

Fay Wentworth
  The Scavenger   81

Kathryn Moss
  Fall   87
  Evolution   87
  Slugs   88
  Sudden Psalm   89
  The Queen of the Summer   89

Sue Wood
  Hey-ho said Roly   91

Chris Kinsey
  An Introduction to
    County Mayo   95
  Wind Chill Factor   96
  Breach of the Peace   97
  Seeing Yellow   97
  The Night Before Full Moon   98

Leonie Smith
  Congratulations on Purchasing
    Your Brand New Man   99

Sean Burn
    dante in the laundrette   103
    mayday   104
    history lessens   104
    trans pennine   105
    24:12   106

Karin Bachmann
    A New Beginning   108

Gordon Hodgeon
    In the Purse   112
    Freeze   112
    Circular   113
    Zero   114
    Notice   115

Ruth Henderson
    That to Odin   116

Daphne Rance
    Mrs Linden   123
    The Woman in a Red Dress   123
    City Street in Spring   124
    Studying the Architecture   125
    Nowadays   126

Josephine Fagan
    Venus on a Soap Dish   127

Graham Clifford
    Stealing Summer   131
    Skinned   132
    What I Wrote   132
    The Best Poem Ever Written   133
    What I Really Want To Do   134

Sally Zigmond
    A Twisted Thread   135

Joan Michelson
    Shield   141
    Second Anniversary   141
    Christmas Crow   142
    The Last Week   143
    Brief Bliss   144

Tom Bryan
    Sister of the Sun   145

Derek Adams
    Wreckers   150
    Icarus in the 21st Century   150
    A Century ago   151
    Kite   151
    Prey   152

Tania Casselle
    Like Getting Caught in the Rain   153

Elizabeth Tate
    Retreat   159
    In the Mean Time   159
    Winter Landscape   160
    Relic   160
    Netted   161

Chris Turner
    Elizabeth French's Irrational Fear of Chocolate   163

Tom Bryan
    Road Man   170
    Kitchen Rat   170
    My Mantelpiece   170
    Rush Hour   171
    January Night, Selkirk   171

Maurice J. Ryan
    Mountain Interlude   172

Mike Marqusee
    Aesthetic   177
    The Cat in the Hat   177
    Old Mose Knows   178
    Apologia with Muttered Aside   179
    Song of the Besieged   180

Morag Hadley
    Immortelle   182

Bernadette Cremin
    Art Work   189
    Susan   189
    Thin Curtain   190
    Quarry Tiles   191
    High Ceiling   191

Owen Dwyer
    Greed   192

Short Biographies   196

Judges' Comments

What a blistering day for undertaking the final judging of a poetry competition.

Yesterday, I started in earnest – sifting, reading and re-reading sitting out on the lawn outside my house. I evaluated; constructed hierarchies; ended up with six piles of A4 paper. The west wind that was threshing the huge horse chestnut trees and cooling me down kept whispering suggestions in my ear.

Today it was too warm to concentrate outside so I spread manuscripts around a room and lounged with them as I adopted various positions, from horizontal to vertical, till it was time to cut to the chase and make final decisions – choose which number (there were no names) had won.

In the end, it was easy for me to pick number 115 – that turned out to be Sue Vickerman's poems. I love their precision and accumulation of detail; the beating heart in them, which is expressed both as rhythm and purpose; the lightness of touch; the surprise.

"Meanwhile, on a rock cling-wrapped in jelly-fish,
a solitary shag lands in a shallow glide, his posture
less refined than a cormorant, his loosely-crested nape
spiked, rakish, brave against the dashing water

and I noticed him looking me over in a way you never do."

(The sensitively thin bill of the shag)

I also enjoyed the particular *salt-lick* of the world that accrued when I read the poems together. Edgy, elemental, tender, they help me to understand more about what it is I'm doing, being human. I'm really looking forward to reading the collection.

I chose another three poets for commendation: Joan Michelson, Gordon Hodgeon, Mike Marqusee.

I love Gordon Hodgeon's vigour and singularity, the way particulars become universals without any straining. The poems have their feet on the ground and their hearts and heads in the skies. They have the confidence to not over-explain. I love *Freeze*. It cooled me down. Made me shiver and my ears tingle.

I appreciated Joan Michelson's breadth of poetic form, and his/her delicate exploration of loss. *Shield* stands out for me, ending with the exquisite "Words/like moths opening/their wings."

Mike Marqusee's poems, with their great titles, took me somewhere else. I especially like the *Cat in the Hat* whose world Wallace Stevens' mind would feel at home in.

I won't mention any other individual poets or poems, other than to say *Well Done!* if you got into the anthology. If you didn't, don't let it put you off. Keep going!

Now the sun's falling out of the sky. The only sensible thing for me to do after such a sweltering and sedentary day is to mow the lawn, my head filled with the fire of all your images and rhythms. Thanks.

Subhadassi (Walton, July 2003)

Almost every day I hear someone's story, they cover every aspect of human life and emotion. These stories are real, so how can I judge a fictional writing competition? That was the question I posed myself when asked to do so. Well, one thing I do is read. I read a lot and have done so all my life, also I'm more than familiar with human emotions and the feelings that always go with a good story.

When I got the stories to read I wasn't disappointed. The diversity of styles and the sheer quality of work made the process a pleasure. I don't want to pick out any one in particular, as I think the final judgement is such a close call. Suffice to say, I was thrilled with the variety of subjects tackled. The ability to tell a story, convey an emotion, a feeling or tell a joke was of the very highest standard. I hope you find this anthology as much of a pleasure to read as I did in helping put it together. To all those included, and those not included, Thank You!

Peter Lister

At its best, the short story is a joy and there is joy aplenty here. Once again the standard of stories submitted for the Biscuit competition has been high. It makes judging incredibly dificult but provides riches for the reader. Enjoy!!!

Denise Robertson

Foreword

The Biscuit competition is now established as an annual event on the international literary scene. It is not the biggest competition in terms of numbers of entries, but that means the intake is manageable and all work is thoroughly read. Neither does it offer the highest prizes, but it does offer publication alongside prize monies. And it promises to publish, it does not tease with the idea. See the catalogue list on our website. Launched in 2000, Biscuit has already published seven titles – three poets' collections and four anthologies – providing a total of one hundred and twenty writers' works published. By the end of 2004 it will have published a further seven books: an anthology, three novellas and three poetry collections.

Biscuit now has Arts Council of England (North East) funding. That surely signals an endorsement of Biscuit's credibility. The money provides for publishing three new writers (quite apart from those emerging directly from the competitions): two poets' collections and a novella or collection of short fiction.

Why novella, indeed why short fiction? Be assured, it is not because they are cheaper to print. Biscuit supports literary works. The novella, of 25K to 40K words, utilizes very much the same tightly composed, minimalist form as the short story. Both require the skilled composition of heightened language and economy of words; very similar in fact to the art of poetry. That is why they sit side by side in this anthology.

At its best, short fiction, like poetry, is a magnificent art. Yet here in the UK, it is sidelined. Short stories and novellas, particularly the former, are marginalized by the mainstream publishing industry. And that includes the literary agents. Short fiction is being ostracized to extinction. Almost. Thankfully, there is now a movement fighting to save the form. *The Save Our Short Story Campaign* is underway right now, led by ACE North East and writer Val McDermid (see www.saveourshortstory.org). Publishers like Biscuit are doing their bit too.

But why do we have this situation? Why is short fiction being sidelined by mainstream publishers? The answer is obvious; it doesn't sell enough copies to make money. Putting that another way, the public – and that means you and me – is not buying the books when they are offered. And why not? The answer to that is less obvious, but this writer has a sneaking feeling that writers themselves are to blame; and they are starting to realize it. The word "accessible" has lately entered the art world's vocabulary. Could it be that a fairly recent school of writers has pitched its work at such a high academic level it has excluded the general reader? And can that apply to poets too, because poetry sales are in just as low a state? Can it be that writers have been expounding far too much energy on writing for fellow writers? Literary narcissism, gazing longingly at its own reflection in the lake, finally drowning in an attempt at sexual consummation? Art looking inwards upon itself, contemplating its own navel? So what's to do about it? We should not, will not, dumb down the work. What we can do, surely, is maintain academic standards and still provide an entertaining read. Making the work accessible. Accessible to the public readership. That is Biscuit's belief, and that is why it employs both "academic" and "lay" readers to judge the competition entries. This writer has an MA in creative writing, but is not an intellectual; he just knows a good read of fiction and poetry when he sees it. And he played a part in judging the Biscuit entries. So did Subhadassi, who is a freelance poet, and so did Peter Lister, who is a police detective. And so did Denise Robertson, who is a best-selling novelist and agony aunt. A heady mix there, would you agree?

Biscuit entries this year arrived from all parts of the United Kingdom. There were also entries from the United Arab Emirates; Switzerland; Sicily; France; Ireland; Jersey; Hong Kong; Australia; yet oddly enough all of those were in the short story category; poets were wholly British – and Irish. So much then for the death of the short story; it seems to be still strongly alive around the world. And here's a thing; I am informed that the short story is not just alive but thriving and strong in USA and Eastern Europe. By thriving, I take that to mean, such books are available in the bookshops and people are buying them in decent quantities. So what's wrong in the UK? I would suggest that the answer can be found in the reading of contemporary North American literary fiction, short and long. We can learn a lot from the Alice Munros and Raymond Carvers *et al* across the Atlantic. And by the reading of Biscuit authors' works. Unless of course, you know better?

Brian Lister

2003 First Prize Winners
Fiction: Tracey Fuller
Poetry: Sue Vickerman

Previous First Prize Winners
Fiction:
Ruth Henderson   2001
Veronica Lloyd   2002

Poetry:
Chris Preddle   2001
Bob Beagrie   2002

Patrons
Denise Robertson
Katrina Porteous

If you would like details of how to enter Biscuit fiction and poetry competitions, or a list of publications, please send sae to:
Biscuit Publishing Ltd.
PO Box 123
Washington
Newcastle upon Tyne
NE37 2YW

e-mail: info@biscuitpublishing.com

www.biscuitpublishing.com

Sue Vickerman
The Sensitively Thin Bill of the Shag

A squabble in the eaves, housemartins,
wakes us early. As I pour your breakfast tea
a gannet flop-glides off the lighthouse,
drops between smoke-rings of mist

while you swill spit from the basin,
put in your contacts, peer out at the tide
already lapping the slip-way, and I know
that you're going to shout *Heron! Let's go down.*

At the edge, where bladder-wrack stretches
skin-tight on the knees of boulders, where my boots
flatten pods and pick up slime, I remark
that the tide will isolate us if we're not careful

but you stride on, as usual, over thick kelp stipes,
shadows of fish in pools, liver-fleshed anemones,
and straddle the thin smile of a ravine, disregarding
the sea, how it foams your trainers into a wet shave,

how oyster-catchers clack their knitting-needle beaks
like wives complaining, and herring gulls line up,
laddish, on ledges. Your interest is only in exotic visitors.
Whinchat you call over wave-noise. *Or maybe a wheat-ear.*

Meanwhile, on a rock cling-wrapped in jelly-fish,
a solitary shag lands in a shallow glide, his posture
less refined than a cormorant, his loosely-crested nape
spiked, rakish, brave against the dashing water

and I notice him looking me over in a way you never do.
Steep-browed, thin bill; fine hook at the tip. When I skid,
blushing, on mustard-smeared granite, he winks,
shows me his profile, flexing his seaweed wings.

Trelleborg to Sassnitz

The radar of a small green lighthouse is spinning
across my porthole. You beckon me out to the deck, point
at a tousle of windmills on the headland as we dock
alongside the dark sinew of somewhere that isn't Dover,
the unwinding snake of another foreign territory.

Sue Vickerman

In the phone-booth of the terminal, I clutch the faint question
in the receiver, picking with difficulty through currency
in your uncurling fist. Salt-lipped, you shift your rucksack
while the digital seconds flicker out, and my answer
no we're not in Berlin; not yet, gets cut to a single negative.

Waiting for Puffins

You said they would arrive in May.
Noticing a gossamer of droppings
cobwebbed over the cliffs, sheer rock
feathered into a duvet, my hopes soar
out of the window. I forfeit a cooked breakfast
for seaweed and scrambled pudding-stone,
locking the lighthouse but leaving a note
just in case: *Gone to puffins. You know where.*

Scanning the chess-board of sleek-backed auks
I train your loaned binoculars on profiles,
rubbing the steam of my hot look from your lenses,
trying to catch a distinctive beak, curious
eye-markings, tell-tale red among the grey suits
of kittiwakes. A thick-set fulmar hangs stiff-winged
on an updraught, stalls, then drops. Guillemots,
startled, unfurl overhead. I dodge, umbrella-ed.

*Auks need ledges on which to rest, whereas puffins
dig burrows in the soft ground of cliff tops.*

My boots catch on lichen, slip in pools
while the rising tide pulls slowly at the time
available, slides round another inlet. I clamber
beyond common sense, sure of a sighting,
the distinctively large head, the amusing waddle.
Scaling the milk-stained cliff among the waterfalls
of nests, I reach the final outcrop, and discover
an inaccessible bay, curved in a lipless smile.

There! I zoom in, breathless, on a patch like liquorice,
touching the focus lightly, waiting for a profile
that doesn't jab and point. I blink back salt,
blink away my double-vision, a thousand couplings.
But there are no bright, calypso beaks, jolly as plastic;
no sad-eyed, comical sea-birds from book-spines
and cartoons, the ones you promised; only auks'
dark looks and razorbills' blunt chins, and my eye-
corners lapped by the encroaching edge of the sea.

Sue Vickerman

Skylark

A shaken-out blanket of yellow rape
makes us pull up, picnic-minded. I laugh
as a comic-strip hare bounces into a field
nippled with cut turnips, but you miss it

and then on our backs in the rumpled meadow
I hear it first: the spiralling phrases,
the rising hover of the classic aerial singer,
piece of grit swimming over my eyeball,
a flicker in the chlorine sky. *Look*
I indicate the particle against the sun,
the speck on the blue screen of August

but you find the skylark sharp-tongued, shrill
as a kettle, its vibrato making you shiver,
sanding your sockets like migraine,
its ultimate plunge splitting your head.

Stonehaven Harbour

We could do that. But your dark glasses look,
instead, out to sea. I say *Maybe*. The yacht-clubbers
on the slip-way zip each other into black rubber
then step nimbly, suction-soled, banana-skinned,
onto perspex. Their silhouettes link, seamless
then part, like mime artists, dodging the swing of the sail.

Taking my ice-cream from you I feel it again,
the bullet-sized piece of knowledge triggered
by my reaching arm; the small knot of fear
in my breast, 'non-urgent,' assigned to the slow list.
We float by the Marine Hotel, the Ship Inn,
a backpack laid out on the harbour wall, hikers
from Germany, a gang of over-sixties friends.
White sails kite over the water; a child complains;
the golden retriever swims slowly back to base
with the stick. Waiting is hardest at weekends.

Tracey Fuller

The system was turned on

"The radiators were noted to warm up in a reasonable degree of time. The radiators are the pressed steel type. They are served by small bore painted pipes, presumably copper."

I stand in the upper room overlooking the bay. The gulls and cormorants, not to mention shags, perch on the wooden posts in the water. They flap their wings, dive arrow sharp and disappear in the swirl. The window is mottled and the sea swings in the glass and hangs there. When I move it sways, like a sea shanty.

"There are softer red bricks forming the segmental arches over the openings. One or two of these have eroded. There are concrete subsills. Part single skin. A cement plinth that is partly off key. There is dampness internally. The knob handle is loose."

I smooth my palms over the plastered walls feeling for dampness, feeling for cracks. I turn with a start but you are not there, how could you be. You will have heard of course about the house. The usual family grapevine working its way, threading through the back to back streets. Better than the whispers in alleyways of last month. You will hear that the house is a long way from you and that I will not be able to visit often. Scotland's west coast is a tricky place to get to and a tricky place to leave. You will hear, no doubt, that I am happy to be going, that work and my life have moved on and that the temporary move back to the bosom of the family could never work out for a career woman who needs to keep pace with her work. There are flights, of course, but they don't land within a hundred miles of you and with the winter setting in it is easier to stay put. You'll be pleased for me I'm sure, when you meet the other family members, the wives drinking coffee and laughing over the kids, you and the lads leaning against the wall talking about your golf handicap or the funny thing that your youngest did on the range. Someone will mention it, the move so sudden, so unexpected; when they thought I was settling in so well. Of course, they never expected me to come back in the first place. What on earth was there for me in a place like that? Nothing but small town, no culture, no work to speak of, no friends, only family. Just family. Why would I, who have been away so long, want to go back?

"The main rear elevation windows are sash type, there is a missing sash cord, some flaking paint."

I run my fingers over the white paint; it creeps in under my nails. Outside the pier curls into the water, a boat appears from around the headland. From here, I can see nothing before Iceland.

"There is some flaking paint to the bargeboard and there may be some minor wet rot."

I remember the rot setting in; probably when I was around six or seven and you were say nine or ten. Playing in the fields, kicking through leaves. Bows and arrows, catapults. Mudslides we made down the side of a bank at the bottom of our grandmother's garden. We slid down the slide until the mud spread all over our clothes, oozed through our fingers. You tried to push mud down my t-shirt, I rubbed my hands through your hair until it stuck up in brown spikes. We filled our shoes with it and squelched around feeling it slip between our toes. We ran headlong through nettles to the broken furniture at the bottom of the garden, climbed the fence and ran through the field screaming like our Gran's kettle, twirling our arms like sycamore helicopters. Running back, mouth open, I ran headlong into the washing line. It caught me through the mouth slick cut like a fish with twine in its gills. You stopped running. The others, for there were always others, carried on. You came back and held my wrists as I shook with shock, blood running with mud. I would have spat it out but my lips were open and gaping. Too sore to move, my mouth filled with blood.

There was chicken for tea. Everyone tucked in. I sat by the fire. You would not eat to keep me company.

"Over the porch there is a small-hipped roof, the rain water pipe is shared, it discharges to a gully in the front path."

The rain for those two weeks in August wouldn't stop; booked on purpose to ruin things I was sure. But looking at pictures we always seem to be brown, even in black and white you can tell, there's a silky sheen to our skin. The minute the sun split the sky we were off to the beach, me in bikini bottoms with a little white pleated skirt attached. No top. You probably couldn't get away with that today.

I watch from the window, a small child and her mother muffled in scarves walk carefully down the stone steps to the shingle beach beyond the pier. The child stoops to pick up a shell and waves it at her mother. I remember us paddling and rootling in rock pools, digging interminably long ditches to re-direct the stream that ran from the hills onto the beach. We always ended up smothered in sand, throwing it and rolling in it and rubbing it into each other's skin.

"There are brick copingstones and lead soakers at the abutment."

I walk around the house and peer out of the window, tracing my finger along a diagram, twisting the report around to see what they are talking about. Downstairs the estate agent is chatting to the owner; I can hear them in the kitchen, glasses chinking.

Tracey Fuller

You had the glasses lined up. I was under-aged so you had to get them, what was it Pernod and black? You wanted to drink snakebites but thought Carlsburg was more mature. I wore a purple jump-suit, with all the zips and had my hair plaited like Boy George. We danced insanely to the Boomtown Rats and The Jam and argued about Paul Weller. There was some confusion and a fight, there was always a fight, and we stumbled out with tables and chairs flying, laughing. You always tried to get me to drink too much, ordering doubles, lining them up. I never did.

I wonder at you now, you hardly touch a drop, just a couple with the lads after a round. Not too many, you're driving and there are often the kids to pick up.

I pull down the loft ladder.

"Are you okay up there?" the agent shouts up the stairs peering round the banisters. There is laughter from the kitchen, he doesn't venture too far or wait for an answer but heads back to the kitchen and the vendor. I don't know why he's here, except that he'll be sorry when this house is sold. He must love me as a client, with all my questions, gives him lots of opportunity to pop by. He pays a lot of attention to his customers, well this one at least.

I gingerly step onto the loft ladder and up into the void above.

"The slates are on battens on an undercloak of sarking felt. The joists run from front to rear. There are pole plates forward and rear. The joists pass under these. The rafters are notched over."

I notched up a few friends pretty quickly. It was best for you, I suppose, when I didn't know anyone. You had a certain amount of power then. Once I knew people I flaunted it a bit. I wasn't just the girl visiting in the holidays. I didn't need you to take me out any more. I remember dancing. I knew you were watching me, leaning on the bar. A thread ran between us. I brushed past you. You grabbed my arm. "Dance with me." I laughed, flouncing my homemade ra-ra skirt, I thought I was Bananarama. Later, you still drinking, me slumped on a sofa, "Come home with me," you whispered, or was it slurred. "Leave them and come home with me." I wish I had. Maybe none of this would have happened.

A christening wasn't it? Children running everywhere, cold buffet, those curling sandwiches, everything with egg or sausage meat. Our cousin drunkenly persuading me that I looked great and I'd grown up a stunner. You raising your eyes to the ceiling, me balancing on my stool, smiling, waiting for him to go. He did, of course, as they always did. It was as if we had some kind of people-repellent spray that kept them away. Or blinded them if they were there. The invisible line between us reached half way round the world. Reached as far as a beach in Queensland when I felt you tug it and I came spinning back. Spinning back to this rocking barstool.

I ripped up beer mats. You ran your hands over your bottle of Bud. My finger traced the round top of my wine glass. You seemed to have picked up a woman from somewhere; she wouldn't unhook her arm from your neck. She had you in her shepherd's crook but I was Little Bo-Peep. My sheep were scattered and long gone, I needed help to find them. I excused myself and headed outside, you followed. You seemed to have detached her, your body thudded into mine as the children screamed on the bouncy castle.

"The purlins do not bear to the flank walls. They are supported on timber corbels, brick corbels and short struts. The latter partly bear on the wishbone chimney flue."

It was at that wedding, do you remember? Of course, how could you forget? It was your wedding. The photographs taken, she seemed to be scowling in them, the photographer couldn't get a decent smile out of her. I moved away and she seemed to relax. Her funny puffy white dress and funny puffy white face. I danced with everyone that night, I don't normally dance at weddings but I really let myself go. She seemed to spend most of the time in the lounge area away from the dance floor getting more and more drunk. I suppose I should have gone home early, that would have been the honourable thing to do but our thread kept me there. You leaning on the bar, kissing the aunties, swinging the children round, leading a conger and then quickly leaving them to it to meet me on the lawn. The whole wedding party looped its way round the chairs and tables, knit one purl one, stitching up the room into a tight closed ball. Shrieking, deaf to the muffled sighs outside.

"There is a screeded area outside the kitchen, there is a wooden trellis and an arch, there is a small wooden felt shed. The garden requires some attention."

So it continued with me moving back, the line between us too great to bare the constant tugging and stretching. It seemed to be fine for a while, the magic we wove managed to keep the prying eyes and wagging tongues at bay. The babies I sat on my hip and swayed while she had a night off and you did some work on the electrics/plastering/woodwork. I can't remember. She knew of course. She knew from the start, she knew before we did. But the others didn't and they dragged her out for her nights with the girls. "They're cousins, leave them alone they're fine. What do you think they're going to do? Have an affair?" They hooted with laughter at the thought. We laughed the loudest and longest.

"Water was run from the various fittings, no blockages noted."

Tracey Fuller

The blockage came in the guise of one of your girls, mop haired and sleepy tumbling out of bed to the sound of us.

"Making the bed darling, that's all, go back to sleep."

But she had seen the sheets strewn, your tools scattered on the floor, street lamps showing enough. You talked it through with her, laughed it off in your cavalier way. Asked me when I was babysitting again. I applied for a transfer to the Glasgow office.

The little boat struggling round the headland has made its way into the harbour and the fishermen are lugging off their catch. The girl and her mother have collected their shells and are trudging back up the steps. I push up the loft ladder and close the hatch. Downstairs the giggling has hushed. It's evening, and you will be picking up the kids from their child-minders and planning the night ahead. You will have heard by now and when they tell you I am gone you can act in real surprise. You will not need to fake it.

With thanks to Nigel Enever for an inspiring structural survey.

Lee Morris

Female Study I: On the Scent

There is a row of unopened boxes
in your bathroom cupboard,
each one with an exotic-sounding name
and a beautifully-shaped bottle
of perfume,
presumably because people think
they are a fitting gift
for a girl like you –
an it-girl without the sniffy attitude,
a babe without the bland bitchiness –
and presumably because
they can imagine
all five-foot-ten of you
in a sweaty two-piece
hurtling down a desert dune,
or your fine-boned hands
resting on the handlebars of an old bicycle,
choosing a mixed bouquet
for your wicker pannier,
or your brisk civet walk,
as you walk your wolf
with your red coat buttoned up against the cold.
And they don't really care
if the notes are high or low or medium
or floral or fruity
or spicy or musk;
they just know that a mix
of crazy vulnerability,
pretty-blue peekaboo eyes,
well-cut nose,
and earrings that trail your smokey laugh
is entêtante
and hope they just might catch it on the breeze.

Female Study II: Self-portrait

The female runs through her hair
noticing for the first time
the asymmetry of her receding temple.
There is no hiding it.
Attempts to conceal it with a fringe have failed
dismally – the pride of an arching cusp.

The hair is thick and when she dips
her back and brushes it down hard
and shakes it back,
she finds it has a will of its own,
like a half-flayed animal.
It is dry and tindery, like the bush,
and will be for hours now,
recovering. But when it is calm
she will see the lighter streak
that falls, maybe a hundred acres wide,
across the left side of her face.
It has been there since
childhood, when the sun
licked the strands to gold
but even then it was scraped back
almost to the bone.
It is still long enough to taste
and comforting to suck –
a dribble of wild honey in a hot brown bough.

Female Study III: Bernadette

Beautiful Catholic Bernadette,
the contradictory black sheep,
hair like a witch's streak of white,
conception ruled you'd never reach
the obligatory brunette
sung in your sisters' six-part mass.

It was totally inappropriate,
but wholly within character,
for you to flick your fag-ash on the floor
at your bloody-minded father's wake,
rippling the warm after-death tipple,
and drag your boyfriends home from hell,
and trash the positive-thinking books
that kept your mother's faith from fading
like the blooms in the tangled garden
or the sweat-thumbed notes in her purse.
You had the look of her easy prime,
the high-arched brows and marbled skin,
unlike the eighth, who looked as drawn
and tired as her own worn-out skull,
as if the womb now cried 'enough!'
and continuing might produce a corpse.

Lee Morris

Did she notice the holy water spill
when you dangled lightly over the font?
Or did her vision of the gentle saint
distract her from the damp at her feet,
and the stream pushing at the closed church doors
and the river in the bursting street,
that sprawled and fanned to a delta,
where warning bells don't stir the air
and horses breed free, milky young,
where infants curl their toes in the sand
and turn their heads to droplets of sun?

Female Study IV: Babushka

I loved the game, the gentle unscrewing of self,
    the soft creaking of the wood, a regular denuding.
First, the outer shell was cracked, swollen arthritic bones
    snapped
    and by invitation
    we went down to greet the costumed women.

They are clothed as we remember them.
We finger them tenderly,
    descending until my nail can't find a cut,
    until I hold you in my hand, tiny, complete –
    satisfied.
Then when your fantastic ordinary life is arrayed
    like a xylophone for me to hammer out your tones,
    in a dancing line of blinking stones, and just-blossoming jasmine,
    set by girdles inscribed with golden mottos,
    a caravan of chips and cracks,
    a row of innocent eyes and wicked smiles,
    the process in reverse, the smallest doll is covered.

I am careful to complete the formalities, in case it is the last time,
    aligning the hips and the arms,
    until, by gradual compaction, the past is hidden,
    darkened in a pregnant piece, a family toy.

Lee Morris
Female Study V: Glass Eye

I do not want to see you take out your right eye,
    large Afrikaner woman.
Why should you do such a thing to a little child?
I'm afraid of your magic.
My nerves are dangling like thin broken blood vessels.
My mother wants me home now.

Get Lost

Arnie was sweating now. It was happening again, that feeling of deep fear churning his guts and making his head spin. That lousy feeling of being hopelessly lost. And to be lost on this particular night, well that was dumb. Extreme dumb, he said to himself, screwing up his eyes to see through the sheet of rain.

He had sworn to himself that he'd sort this out. A man of thirty three in his own downtown city of goddam Kansas City should not be lost. It had been his one weak spot in a long career of crime, this tendency to take the wrong turn, to trust in memory and not check out the city plan.

"Damn it, that was the junction for the interstate, I could have been real way out of direction there . . . it's this blasted rain. I can't see . . . not a thing."

Arnie felt all the weaknesses come bursting through his mind again. He was carrying too much weight. He was getting short of breath. The last heist had been a close run thing and they only made off with two hundred bucks. Sadie had laughed at him, then it turned sour. As he screeched the old Chrysler round a tight bend, he could hear the conversation again.

"Arnie, I can feed four mouths on eighty bucks? You wanna live on baked beans all next month? Arnie, get a proper job. You're too old for this. It's for a young guy, this dodgy life with the Schmidts . . ." Sadie, her long black curls shaking as she lost her cool, was so beautiful, and he'd let her down so bad . . .

But the Schmidts. Oh God, he was late for the meeting with the Schmidts. They'd crush his privates in a vice, they'd pay a call on his kids in school, breathing threats through the bars. The Schmidts. God, they had no patience. Let 'em down once and you're dead meat. He glanced at the clock. Ten past eight. He was ten minutes late. And he had the papers. He felt the wodge of papers and the plan of the jewelry shop in his inside pocket. Again, he mumbled the address to himself . . . twenty first, east . . . Mario's ristorante . . . twenty first east . . . and he was on, erm . . . Christ! There was a sign for Aichison. He was north. He'd gone damn north. Now the rain was pelting the windscreen like hail.

He would have to ask. It was shameful but he had no choice. He pulled in to a gas station, following the sign. Crawling out of the car, he saw an old guy yanking at a drinks machine.

"Hey, say, friend, I kinda lost my way . . . not been here for some time . . . can you point me towards east twenty first – Mario's place?"

As the guy turned he realised that the face was elsewhere, like gone away for the vacation onto planet nuts. "Sorry . . . I see you're not well . . ." Arnie turned away. But he got a string of abuse.

"Not well, you ain't no idea what I got in my head, you weirdo foreigner . . . why, I got dreams of white lions and a trip to Africa in here. Yessir, I got dreams in colour and you got a punk's crap game. I can see you're a lost cause . . . but my pal Homer can help."

Arnie, now sodden and unable to see anything clearly, glanced to one side to focus on a tall, huge guy with a smile that made your blood turn ice. It took only seconds for Arnie to be in the car and heading away, anywhere, as fast as his heart pumped.

Mel was wiping the counter again, for the tenth time in that hour. It was hard, coping with the work in the diner while carrying little Dean. It was going to be a boy, and the boy was going to be Dean, after Jimmy. But boy was it a chore that night. Not one customer except old Prof. Deneyer, the cookie loner. He was muttering poems into his chocolate drink in a corner, and Mel was singing to herself, then running down her top ten films, then taking a few dance steps . . . anything to stave off the boredom. She took to talking to Jimmy, rubbing her belly and saying, "Little Jimmy Caborn, you are gonna have a life, I mean a LIFE . . . not some bum rap like your ma got, nor the life of a grease monkey like your daddy. No, you are gonna be a mover and a shaker and kick some ass, my son . . . you hear?"

She caught sight of herself in the long mirror by the coffee machine and, moving in close so she could inspect her skin and her smile, she whispered, "Not bad for a young mom . . . you're wearing well, girl... just keep on hanging in there, Melanie . . ." She saw the blonde hair across her face, the slightly plump red cheeks and the mascara, maybe a little too strong. But the eyes, they were her strongpoint. Like Gina Lollobrigida her pop had said once . . . Then, from the corner of her eye, she saw the little plump guy come in, wet like he'd swum across the road. He flapped his hat dry and emerged from his trenchcoat with a gasp and a flutter, eventually finding a high seat by the bar and groaning.

"Wet I guess?" Mel said, trying for a smile.

"You a comedian? Get me a coffee . . ."

"A smile don't cost, fella."

"Tonight, you'd have to crank a crease in my face with a jack."

"That bad huh? Here's a coffee . . . real strong to set you up."

He sipped it and wrapped his hands around the mug, then dipped his head as if about to weep.

"Hey, look, it ain't that bad, nothing's that bad. Don't crack up on me." Mel touched his neck gently.

He looked up and stared at her. "Miss, you're looking at the definition of failure. Arnie Short. Failed clerk, failed salesman and now . . . failed man. A bum husband and father, no hoper . . . and why? Cos he can't master the geography of his home city . . ."

"Hey that's not so bad. I get lost every time I visit my sister in Lincoln, and that's three times a year!"

"But I'm talking business. I mean, I just had to turn up for a . . . a business meeting and, well, good old Arnie, lost again! You know what my friends call me – Scenic Route! Yeah, Scenic Route Short. In my business that's so bad . . . I mean, in my line of work you get monicas like Scarface, The Fist, Blade, the Sicilian . . . but me, I'm not even 'Shortie' – I'm Scenic Route. I always take the long way round and get lost some place . . . another coffee Miss."

"Call me Mel. And this is Dean in here." She patted her belly and smiled. Arnie was nervous, but a quick look down at her bump somehow brightened him.

"Say . . . I got two kids, just three and six . . . when's he due Miss?"

"Any day . . . officially in three days. They may induce . . ."

Arnie asked permission to feel the bump, and coyly, tapped on her. They both smiled and Mel giggled. "It's my first. My man told me I shouldn't be workin' but well, we sure need the dough. He gave in after I promised him a new CD player with the overtime pay. I've had a few gripes tonight . . . the kid's letting me know he wants out."

Arnie shuffled over to a seat offering a bit more comfort. "Say, it's quiet . . . get yourself a drink and sit with me here, Mel. I need some company."

"Well, you're not one of my regulars are you? Should I trust a stranger." She turned to the Prof. and shouted, "What do you reckon Prof – should I sit with this man?"

"Ah leave me alone woman!"

She explained that the old man was not living in the modern world. "But he's written ten books . . . you wouldn't think the man was a doctor would you, to look at him?" She laughed, and enjoyed thinking about the old man, a regular she knew well.

"No . . . but I bet he knows the way home!" Arnie drank some more, then looked disconsolately down at the melamine table-top, then squeezed some ketchup out, like a bored kid.

"So tell Auntie Mel . . . what's the problem?" She followed her words with a sigh.

"Ah, you hear the tales of misery every night in this place . . . I mean it's a throwback to nineteen seventy! Who owns this place?"

"My Uncle Zack. He's away on his Harley in California just now . . . I stand in. Course I got security . . . in the back"

"A big guy with a cleaver?"

"No, a little guy with a large German Shepherd . . . not near the food, I hasten to add!"

"Well, my problem is simple Mel . . . I should be at a meeting right now with two guys called Schmidt built like armoured cars and with tempers like sore-assed grizzlies. They wanted me to be there. I am not there . . . hence I am history."

Arnie suddenly became aware that Mel was not really concentrating on taking in his life-story. She was wheezing and gasping and grabbing her gut. "Oh for Chrissake, I think I got the contractions getting more severe . . . Where's my husband when I need him? Hey, Arnie, I reckon this is the real thing . . . ARNIE! HELP!" She slumped down to the floor.

Arnie panicked. He yelled at the old man. "Come and help . . . you're a doctor, right?"

"What . . . what's wrong with you . . . you a crook?"

Arnie had to grab him by the collar. "Prof . . . you got to help."

"He's a Doctor of Philosophy, he's no damn use!" Mel screamed.

Then the dog in the back started yapping and a little man with short sight and a stutter popped out to ask what was wrong. He was foreign and had trouble with English.

"Miss Melanie, you in t . . . trouble is right I think, how I help?"

"Arnie . . . drive me to the Mercy Hospital . . . you know . . ."

"Er, Mercy Hospital . . . oh yeah, next to the Wallmart . . . Yeah, I know, I KNOW!"

After being carried to the car by the Prof and the cook, Mel, wrapped in several old coats, was stretched out on the back seat while Arnie put his foot down.

But it was still raining and very dark. He managed to follow some neon lights, after recognizing the Budweiser one. But then, on the next block, everything looked the same again. Just tall brown buildings or lines of stores in semi-darkness. And she was moaning in pain on his back seat.

It was a case of fighting off the panic. Never before had he exercised such self-discipline. One half of his mind looked for the blurred street-signs and the landmarks. The other half issued orders, gave comforting noises and generally tried to recall his own experience of being around at a birth.

"My God, Arnie, I think it's . . . I mean Jimmy's on his way . . . Aaaaargh"

"Melanie, now hold on . . . breathe, breathe, count to six and then deep breath. Now there's a sign . . . Mercy Hospital . . . thank the God of Hoods . . ."

"Hoods? You a hood, Arnie? Never . . . Aaaargh!"

It seemed to last hours, that drive. Then, after a few wrong turns, he found himself staring at a whole bunch of white coats and folks jumping in and out of ambulances. Arnie stopped, not caring where the car was, and yelled for a white coat to come. It took only minutes to wheel Mel into the right place for some help, and she was zooming towards the birthing rooms.

"You the father Sir?" he was asked.

"Ah no, just a friend."

"Wait there . . . ring the father."

Then it was all gone from him, the stress, the noise, the blather of it all. He found himself moving from the chaos of all that human traffic by the vestibule, with the hell of the night streets booming in, to a quiet corner by a coffee machine. He sat down, checked the time. Almost ten. The meeting would be over now. Would they be looking for him? He picked up a magazine and decided to hide behind it. He was reading about the wild west and staying as cool as possible. Then he realised he hadn't rung home. Sadie would be mad as hell. He fumbled in every pocket, feeling for his mobile. Nowhere to be found. It must be in the car. Then he remembered that the car had been left somewhere, anywhere, probably not in a legitimate parking spot. Then, from the depths of his soul, a huge sigh rose, and he had a feeling of soft, accepting resignation before Fate. "Okay Arnie boy, you messed up again. The car is probably in the pound, the wife ready to beat you to pulp. Just read the magazine."

It was a short while after he heard a familiar voice. It was edged with concern and desperation. "Is he going to die, Doc? Is my brother gonna die? Am I gonna die? Just give me the facts?" It was the voice of a Schmidt. It was unmistakably Big Brother Hal Schmidt and he was clearly in some pain.

"Your brother might not pull through, but we're giving it our best shot, Sir." It was that voice of false reassurance that meant, no way, he's dead as a can of catmeat. Then Arnie's heart thumped beats up into his throat as he heard, "It was that loony Arnie, he got the friggin' plan. They wanted the plan . . . is all!"

Arnie felt himself flush red and his ears burn. Then he felt in his inside pocket and there was the plan of the jeweller's place. Bottom line was, his sense of direction had saved his skin.

Peeping out from the magazine, Arnie saw it was a conversation taking place on a trolley. He followed it discretely and saw it enter an elevator on the way to theater. He gave up the chase and wandered back towards safety, past a line of small rooms and busy medics. It was only when he bumped against something hard that he looked down and took in a hard fact. It was a fact given by a little label tied around a solid squat toe. The name was easy to see: Schmidt, Joseph. Oh Christ, it was all up with Arnie Short. He ran for the door.

Sure he was right: in the black night out there, no Chrysler was in sight. An official guy in dark blue garb approached him. "I believe that was your vehicle Sir . . . we had to impound it. Rules is rules."

"I understand . . . I know you have a job to do."

"Well, the good news is, that lady had a little boy. Think you ought to go see her."

Arnie did go in, and Mel was asleep. But the staff let him stare at the kid who was lying in a sort of mini space capsule.

"Well Jimmy Dean. Best advice is, stay clean and never follow the scenic route. In your life, son, go straight from A to B. Ooh, and always hand over the documents. Then you won't end up in the awful situation of sitting in a maternity ward, praying that a German guy upstairs will not recover from his operation."

But there was a sense of a shadow over him, a feeling that he was being watched. A voice from the half-light said, softly like a shrink: "So you're Arnie Short . . . well, we need a driver . . . and one with a plan of a certain jewelry store would be ideal . . . And by the way, you did good tonight . . . my blasted diplomas were no good in an emergency, right? But I had my eye on you . . . you're a nice guy."

"The Prof?" Arnie turned.

"Yeah, we need a driver. I understand you got experience, Mister Scenic Route Short?"

"Sort of . . ."

"You seem to do well under pressure, so we'll give you lots of that. By the way, the other kraut died. We fixed that."

Arnie whispered to little Jimmy, "He brings one and he takes one, the Good Lord. Welcome to a confusing world, kid."

Doreen Hinchliffe

In Café Picasso

The air is heavy, thick,
redolent of smoke from cigarettes
that down the years
has wreathed its way
through rainy afternoons.
They sit alone, as usual,
killing time beneath a dingy light,
Harlequin and Columbine
eking out their wine
until the clowns arrive
to mark the interval.

Her mouth curved once into a smile
but that was years ago
before life set it permanently
in this narrow line.
Both stare into the distance
gaze beyond the smoke.
She's thinking of a ringmaster –
how she curled his hair
around her little finger,
sure that love would last.
He's thinking of sawdust –
tiny shavings
clinging between the toes
of the fire-eater's daughter
who amused him for a while.

They did talk once, long since,
their kindred spirits courted danger
on the high trapeze
but that was when the animals were wild
before it all became just horses,
jugglers, acrobats, parades.
Now, they walk in tame procession
in costumes that have faded –
their safety net no longer needed.

Intermezzo

It's one a.m. – in bed, but wide awake,
I'm trapped in a prolonged commercial break.

Doreen Hinchliffe

With intermission popcorn in my throat
I press the menopause on my remote
control, take stock, and pose a host of wild
unending questions, as if I were a child:
Are my symptoms real or in my mind?
Do I want fast forward or rewind?
Am I going through a mid-life crisis?
Is this stiffness in my joints arthritis?
Should I take up jogging or aerobics?
Start a self-help group for aging phobics?
Am I moody, broody or plain mad?
Clinically depressed or only sad?
Should I ask a toy boy for a date?
Dare I make that phone call to RELATE?

Oblivious, you stretch your legs and sigh.
In twenty years you've never wondered why
I've seemed detached, withdrawn, nor do you now.
Your arm across my waist, you tell me how
the way I feel is really nothing strange,
then joke it's what your mother called "the change."
You turn away, return to sleep, leaving
a thousand more unanswered questions breathing
beside the poems of Stevie Smith under
my bedside lamp. I look at you and wonder,
can I find some way in time remaining
to tell you I'm not waxing, dear, but waning?

Trick of Fortune

That summer we were King and Queen of Hearts
clutching youthful passion's royal flush.
For one last time the day before you left

hand in hand we strolled across the moor
pretending it was somehow possible
for Africa and England to be one.

We'd said goodbye to fairy story endings
accepted we could never bridge the gulf
that long colonial history had bequeathed,

never cross implacable divides
of culture, race. This was farewell to hearts.
Each of us belonged to other suits.

Then, in half light, she made her slow approach –
The Ace of Spades, casting her long chill shadow,
her thinning hair as grey as ours is now.

Maybe your smooth black skin attracted her,
perhaps the joker sent her for a laugh
or was she just the next card in our pack?

Seeing the world before us, love in our eyes,
she smiled, donning the guise of frail old woman.
We held our breath, wondering if this was fate.

"Such a lovely couple," she murmured kindly,
"Such a lovely couple you're going to make."
She nodded then, awaiting our response.

That instant we were tempted. Instead of spades,
our cards were clubs, their lucky clovers strewn
on paths where black and white seemed meant to be.

The moment hovered, hung suspended like
the giant sun. We watched the scene play out,
frame us forever in its irony.

We gave no answer. The lady moved away,
but even as she turned, without a word,
we sensed that there could be no going back,

our red of passion would be red of pain.
Silently, we walked into tomorrow
destined, we knew, to hold a different hand.

Happy Ever After

When I wanted to climb up the beanstalk
like Rapunzel you let down your hair
you spun straw to gold in the moonlight
made me castles that floated on air.

You'd leave trails of pebbles like Hansel
so I'd follow wherever you led
I planted a kiss in the starlight
We'll be happy forever, you said.

Doreen Hinchliffe

As I slipped the gold ring on your finger
as I slipped the glass shoes on your feet
the constant tin soldier was melting
and the drummer boy starting his beat.

Rumpelstiltskin attended the wedding
with a couple of wizened old hags
our carriage turned into a pumpkin
and at midnight you left me in rags.

How I wish you had let me down gently
with a wave of your godmother's wand
or put me to sleep for a lifetime
turned me back to a frog in a pond.

How I wish you had left me a giant
or a dragon to swallow me whole,
instead of that poisoned red apple
that can never be cut from my soul.

Things Are Never What They Seem

Things are never what they seem.
Tiny colourless seeds cascade the fuschia
tadpoles stretch then flex their lithe green limbs
puny trembling fledglings launch the kingfisher
caterpillars flutter into wings.

Things are never what they seem.
Round-faced moon assumes a crescent sliver
flat horizons hide a cunning curve
bankrupt stars still scatter all their silver
setting suns disguise the rise of earth.

Things are never what they seem.
Romeo's vows dissolve like Dali's watches
dead-ends masquerade as lovers' lanes
velvet voices purr from flabby paunches
passion pulses through protruding veins.

Peter Bromley

Archaeology

Each day, at the head of the valley, they burned the cattle. The bitter smell was carried on drifts of smoke down the hill and was everywhere. It got into our clothes, into our hair. It reached, I am sure, the village down the valley where it would seep into the memory of the young children. I stood and watched with my father from the gate that leads from our farm to the site being used for burning. It was as far as we were allowed to go. Beyond there, only Ministry officials who were supervising were allowed to pass. Our cattle had already been shot and burned. They caught the disease early on. We were watching other people's cattle being burned now.

"There's nothing left to do," he said.

"We'll get the compensation."

"That's not it," he said, and we turned to retrace our steps back towards the farm, spending several minutes scrubbing the strong disinfectant into our protective footwear. The liquid was thick and yellow. Even through the clothing, we could feel our skin prickle and our eyes water. As my father scrubbed, I looked up and across the hills. There was still some snow on the distant fell tops.

In the kitchen, my mother had prepared lunch. We ate in silence, as we usually did then. There was not much to do on the farm with the cattle gone. Not much to say. Father kept telling us he would buy some more stock when the burning was over. I once asked him why and he simply answered "Because."

The kitchen was always the warmest room in the house. It continued to smell of animals; still smelled of a working farm. The two dogs came and went as normal although we could not let them out across the fields. Our days were spent sitting in the thin light of the kitchen. I would read the newspapers and the farming magazines, my finger running down the pages as I read. If the door opened, the smell of burning came back into the room from off the hill.

We mostly spoke to our neighbours on the telephone, following the spread of the disease through them and the press. My mother's habit was to cut out the important articles and keep them.

I was young when I first discovered her old cuttings. My parents were out and I was looking for hidden Christmas presents. They'd gone to the village for a dance, leaving me with my elder brother. It was him who suggested we look for the presents. He said that they wouldn't be back for hours. I went into their bedroom. I didn't find any presents, but in their tall-boy I found old newspaper articles, they were in a box with other things – tickets for dances, photographs of them when they were younger. There were layers of things she'd kept. Those at the bottom of the box were from a time before my brother and I were even born. I found cinema tickets from the days when the village hall showed films.

There were two tickets with the name of the film hand written on the plain numbered pieces of paper. In the box, I also found articles that told of the last outbreak of the disease. There was a picture of the vans and lorries parked outside the village. Another showed three or four men standing staring at the camera. They were wearing short white coats over their normal clothes. A policeman was close by. These pictures had intrigued me back then. I spent a long time looking at them. I thought about how, in the middle of it all, they'd gone to see a film in the village hall. The tickets nestled snugly between the two photographs and the articles.

My brother shouted from the spare room that he had found the presents, so I tidied up the box, and pushed it to the back of the drawer, where I had found it. The drawers smelled of my parents; of my mother's talcum powder, the smell of my father's jackets and the subtler, older smell of the wood.

There was still meagre work to do on the farm. With the beasts gone, we needed to disinfect the buildings. A few months after our cattle had been burned I started on the barns. I returned one evening from cleaning them, ready for the eventual return of the cattle. My mother was cutting out an article at the kitchen table. I asked her what it was about. She told me to wait until she had finished and that I could read it then. But, I was eager to leave, and before she finished I set off for the village for a drink with my friends. There, in the pub, we fell into the routine of drink. The talk was of the disease, whose farm had it, and how far it had spread. Over a game of pool one of my friends asked.

"How's you brother?"

"OK. Don't hear from him much."

"Has he got a woman?" my friend asked.

"Not that I know of."

"He got out at the right time."

"Too right." I said, as I hammered in the black, the frustration of months released momentarily.

From the back bar, I could hear the sound of the juke-box. As I racked up the balls again and lined up behind the cue-ball, I knew who was in the bar by the music that had been selected. I knew the sequence the tunes would follow.

What routine there was without the cattle numbed us all. At supper one evening, my mother produced the box of cuttings, tickets and articles that normally stayed in their room at the back of the tall-boy.

"You might be interested in this" she said. "It'll give you something to do for a while." I did not want to tell her I had seen much of it when I was younger. I already knew most of its contents. In the tense, illicit silence of their room years ago, I used to read the articles that my mother had cut out of the press. The articles from the local press about the village. The articles concerning our school, sports days, a catalogue from the village show with my name for coming second in some competition. Reading my name back then had set my heart racing. There were articles about the valley where we lived. There was even one from the national press; a faded Sunday supplement that the country would have read. It had filled me with pride to think that everyone had read about our valley.

But not since my brother left had I been back to the box. His going was a fracture in our lives. On the day he left, there was mostly silence in the kitchen. My mother cooked a large full breakfast, trying to joke that it would be the last good meal he would eat for some time. He told them he would write and come back often. His first purchase was going to be a car, he said. The smell of the cooking meat hung deep and rich in the kitchen. There was a clatter of moving crockery and cutlery, but little conversation. About half an hour before my brother left for the bus, my father got up saying that he needed to go and sort out the cattle. The dogs got up instinctively and went to the door as he rose.

"Can't they wait, this morning?" asked my brother.

"No," said my father, and he held out his hand to shake my brother's hand. As their grip slackened, my father turned and picked up his jacket and left.

The box my mother put on the table was still the same one. It was more worn and full to overflowing because of all the additional cuttings. The sides of the box were beginning to bend and tear. It was held together with sticking tape. The order of the collection was still the same though. There were fewer tickets and programmes on the surface, fewer days away from the farm to relieve the work. On the top of the collection was the article she had been cutting out the previous week. I sat at the kitchen table, looking through the box. I was careful not to upset the order of things. I turned up some of the layers that gave me such pleasure when I used to steal into their room. There was a musty smell to these pieces, the paper was brittle and dry. For the first time in many years, I read about the village show, sports days and about my brother's games for the rugby team. I looked through the old photographs of the previous outbreak of Foot and Mouth disease. One faded black and white photograph showed uniformed officials delivering a large container of disinfectant to a farm. Another simply showed the signs that were used to warn people off the land. These made more sense to me now.

And, I read the ageing piece from the Sunday press about our valley. The photograph in the article was taken from the hill opposite. You could see our farm and the buildings clustered around the farmhouse. It was taken before the new metal barn was built. Long before the burning. The article told the history of where we live. The Romans came, mixing with the local tribes. When they left, it was the Vikings. They landed near here, on the coast where the river valley meets the sea. They spread out through the hills, but when they receded, like the tide going out, they left us their own driftwood. In settlement patterns, in hidden timber beneath the ground, but mostly in the names of places. Like in the name of our village, those up and down the valley as well as in the names of the farms and the individual fields. They came and went. And eventually my father farmed the land.

On the farm, the burning has stopped and the land covered over. The buildings have been cleared out and cleaned with disinfectant. We are free to come and go as we please.

I drive my father to the local market. We look at some cattle to replace the ones we lost. The compensation will be through soon and he can start to rebuild his stock. At the market, he casts his eye over all the lots of cattle. He complains that they are a bit thin. He says they are from the south, and too soft for our hills. But he still rubs his hand along their hides and pats them on their thick muscular necks. I remain in the room where they serve tea, sitting with my back against the wall in the corner. There, I listen to the radio and watch him through the windows that look out onto the yards. On the way back, he talks about the other farmers, some of whom he has not seen for several months. He tells me how they have done over the past year. Who is still farming, who is staying in and who is getting out.

As we get back into the house, he takes out the catalogue from the market, and tosses it onto the kitchen table.

"Put that in your collection," he says to my mother. "First auction for nearly a year."

And she picks it up and sets it to one side to put into the top of the box when she goes to bed that evening.

Over supper, I say "I've been thinking . . ."

"What have I told you about thinking?" he says, interrupting, not wanting me to get to the end of the sentence. As I speak, I stare down at the table, moving my hand across its surface, smooth with years of use. I spin the fork round mechanically. I know they are watching me.

"I've been thinking. I won't be following you onto the farm."

The kettle boils, and my mother jumps up, startled, to take it off the hob. She stands it on the draining board and remains standing, facing the range. She moves the dishes and the pans around.

"As you will," says my father eventually.

"What will you do?" asks my mother, turning round from the range.

"I'm going to visit our James."

And, there is no more to be said. My father farms this land and I will not.

I wait for the cattle to return before I go. I help my father get them into the clean sheds. He slaps each one on its side as it passes, and he looks over the shed gate at them for a while after he has penned them in. It is nearly a year since there were cattle here. A week later, I leave.

I drive down the valley towards the main road. It is growing dark, and I switch on the headlights. There is snow, again, on the high fells.

At first, I pass only isolated farms with their inside lights switched on. Further down the valley, I start to pass through the villages. My headlights arc across the village name-plates, each one picked out in the beams of light. As I leave each village, I look in my rear view mirror to look at the sign. I descend the valley, towards the main road leading south. The road is easier to drive now. I can pick up a bit of speed. I drive more quickly, the names of the villages unfurling before me like the pages of a book.

Andrew Neil Blewitt

The Epistles to the Brassicans

Epistle The First
To Brassica Rapa (The Turnip)

O orbèd brassica, I am ashamed
That from the bardic confraternity
There is not one – nor humble nor well-famed –
Who e'en a couplet has addressed to thee.

Full many a bard would oft apply his quill
To hymn the commonplace in yesteryear:
The daisy, buttercup and daffodil –
But wherefore never thee, thou snowy sphere?

Methinks to rhyme thee they all lacked the wit,
And none within a line would hide thy name
Lest by the critics they be soundly smit;
But I, in Shakespeare's form, will thee proclaim,

And rhyme thee, too, in such a style, O Tur
Nip as to gladden e'en the connoisseur.

Epistle The Second
To Brassica Napus (The Swede)

And yet it is not so with thee, O Swede –
That thou art slighted by the bardic breed
And hast not been the subject of a screed
Because of rhymes there be so dire a need.

E'en bards unschooled could not but be agreed
That they no Muse would need to yield a meed
Of rhymes to pen a stave – or ode, indeed;
Yet never theeward doth a poem speed.

That thou art vulgar is't? Of alien seed?
A weed that dwells with worm and centipede
Fit but in byre and mead the kine to feed?
O, piteous 'tis that none hath paid thee heed.

But as it is decreed beyond the Tweed
(Or so we read) – thy weird must aye be dreed.

Andrew Neil Blewitt

Harriss

A sadist
Harriss the head
A hideous stunted sadist

He'd lead morning prayers
(Forgive us our trespasses
As we forgive them . . .)
He'd read the lesson
(Let brotherly love continue . . .)
Then he'd line up the late-boys
And slap their faces
No excuses accepted
Sickness or accident
Snow or dunnosir
He'd slap their faces

Mine included
Many times
And I hated him
For five stinging fuming years
I hated him

His daughter was different
Pretty and properly proportioned
And smiling
Always smiling

Met her at the tennis club
When Harriss and schooldays were history

Dated her once
Nothing special
Just a theatre
Said I'd pick her up

Too late it registered
I could meet Harriss again

And I dithered in her road
And in her drive
And on the doorstep
But I knocked
Eventually

Andrew Neil Blewitt

But it made me late
And he answered the door
And he slapped my face

Never Time to Say Goodbye

I used ter think that when I die
The last I'd say would be goodbye;
I might, if I 'ad time ter spare,
Just add Gawd bless to all those there.
It's not that I'm an 'oly Joe –
It's like the proper way ter go.

Then in the War – the First I mean –
I went ter serve me King and Queen,
But when I got ter fightin' Fritz
I thought I might be blown ter bits
With never time ter say goodbye
Nor kiss-me-'ardy 'fore I die.

Not me nor any other bloke
Could pick the final word we spoke.
Take Jonesey's "bally"; no-one knew
That that was meant for 'is adjoo,
And though it seemed a bloody shame
'e only 'ad 'imself ter blame.

I liked Old Jonesey in a way –
Lieutenant Jones I ought ter say.
'e thought that fightin' wars was fun
And called old Fritzy Boche or 'un . . .
Best edjercated bloke I've known;
'e 'ad a language all 'is own,
With bally this and spiffin' that,
'is sainted aunt, 'is Sunday 'at,
And speakin' Latin just as 'e
Was learned it at 'is mother's knee –
Like when 'e said ter win the war
We 'ad to 'ave this spreedy core.

Well, up at Wipers* we was stuck   *Ypres
In trenches ankle-deep in muck,
And bein' duty-dog that day
'e comes and says "'ow goes the fray?"

I told 'im quiet round about
Though Fritzy 'ad 'is snipers out.
Then up the ladder straight 'e goes;
I warned 'im "'ave a care," Gawd knows,
But out he squints and says all posh
"But I can't see the bally -----"

My Sainted Aunt

Aunt Gertrude was against drink
And moralised Uncle Mort
From affable intemperance
To sobriety and much solemn meditation

But she made no such progress
With Nell her neighbour
Whom she could not persuade by plea or precept
To leave even one room bottle-free

Indeed Nell would urge Aunt
To be like her
Accept St. Paul's advice to Timothy
And take wine for her stomach's sake

Affronted Aunt would refuse
But calling on her after Uncle Mort died
I found specimens about her flat
Of what she'd always called The Devil's Brew

Wine behind the Weetabix
Brandy by the bedside Bible
Friary stout in the fridge
And a bottle of cider beside the lavatory-brush

The wine was for palpitations she said
The brandy for insomnia
The stout was for visitors
And didn't I know cider was an aromatic disinfectant?

It all seemed eminently sensible
Her heart-beat was bold and steady
She slept well
And the fragrance of the disinfectant filled the flat

Andrew Neil Blewitt

And it was typically kind of Aunt
To provide stout for her visitors
Given her firmly-held views
Though I can't recall she ever offered me any

She and Nell spent more time together
With the passing of the years
Though how they resolved their differences over drink
I never knew

The wine served Aunt's heart well
For when she died at seventy-seven
The doctor said it would have beaten longer
Had it not been for the cirrhosis

The Elder Son Speaks Out

"So now he's home again,
And we'd supposed him slain
By virus, thug or beast.
But, father, why a feast?

He's lived with rakes and sots
In questionable spots
(To say the very least)
Throughout the Middle East;

And now, his portion spent,
He plays the penitent
And hourly beats his breast.

So, father, I suggest
Until we know for sure
He'll stay and sin no more
The feast should be deferred."

The fatted calf concurred.

Sue Vickerman

Trekkie

Today must be Monday, as yesterday was definitely Sunday because they were singing hymns on Radio 4. And we moved on a Friday, as it was cheaper to hire the van. I work out, running along my fingers, that I must, therefore, have been at it for seventeen days. Not including the day Mum tried to kill herself.

I sit back on my heels in the miserable green glow of filtered daylight that manages to reach my window through the thick woods outside. I've created an eerie, shadowless place. Almost like being in space.

I'm just assessing what it lacks, those important finishing touches, when Dave knocks at the front door. I know it's Dave: heard his God-mobile bumbling cautiously down the track to our cottage.

I leave him knocking. Let someone else let him in. I've got a paintbrush in my mouth, glue all over my hands, newspaper stuck to the soles of my slippers. Anyway I'm keen to clear up, make it all look perfect, before I receive any visitors. I've entitled this project 'Operation Space Quarters': theming my new bedroom according to my mail-order Star Fleet Communicator uniform. That's the post-2375 uniform (Deep Space 9, the fifth season). The biggest job has been painting the walls and ceiling totally black like the main part of my tunic. I found this big can of black paint in the outhouse when we moved in; the sort you do drainpipes with. Just the job. Shiny.

The uniform I ordered has a red fleece showing at the neck under the zip; consequently I've painted my wardrobe and drawers red. Ideally the bedspread would be red, too. On the neck are the gold pips showing rank. Luckily I had gold model paint left over from when I was into Dungeons and Dragons, which has enabled me to paint my drawer and wardrobe handles gold – and my alarm clock. My second-biggest job was the painstaking work of enlarging the Star Fleet Communicator badge on the left breast of my uniform. This is now done onto the back of an old Man United poster from when I was briefly interested in football, and will go above my bed when the paint's dry.

The tunic's padded shoulders are grey. My computer, when the sheet protecting it from paint is pulled off, deals neatly with the need for a grey element.

Dave's still knocking. Dad must have disappeared outside somewhere after all.

'Coming Dave!'

He won't be bothered. Dave knows what we're like in this family. He'll just be concerned; worried-looking.

'Hi Dave. I was busy upstairs.' Having opened the front door I retreat backwards down the passage towards the sitting room, '. . . just check on Mum. Mum?' I whisper round the sitting room door. 'Are you seeing people?' Dave is wearing his dog-collar so I know he's not on one of his errands to borrow the step-ladder or anything. Must be Mum – a pastoral visit, about her overdose. He's hovering in the passage, looking concerned, like I expected. His wellie boots are clean as a whistle. Mum says they're a statement. Dave hasn't got over the culture-shock of living in the middle of nowhere yet. He describes his manse as 'sinking in a peat bog.' Mum says she's allergic to his Fair Isle sweater. She'll start coughing if he goes in, to make her point.

'How's life, Adrian? Everything alright? Settling in? How's the old asthma?'

'Fine,' I say, a bit irritated by the usual asthma question. It's not like it dominates my life. 'I'm busy on a project' – I hold up my black hands – 'up in my new room. Got to get it perfect. Mum says it counts as educational,' I add hurriedly, as people sometimes look doubtful when I tell them what I spend time on.

I lean into the living room, blocking the entrance until I've had an indication from Mum that she's up to it. She's got that mournful face on, looking in her compact mirror, pulling down the pouches of skin below her eyes. She snaps the compact shut, slips it onto the cabinet that acts as a sort of bedside table, and raises her eyebrows at me in a resigned way which means she's prepared to undergo a visit.

'Is this a good moment, Margaret?' calls Dave apprehensively from the passage.

I move aside, let him through.

'How are you doing? You certainly look more straightened out than two weeks ago!' Dave hovers with his apologetic air in the doorway.

It's true, the living room's spotless; packing crates long gone.

'Has it been so long?' Mum says in a tired voice. 'I've done what I can. Still a lot to unpack upstairs.' She flails weakly with one hand at a pile of TV magazines on the end of the couch where she's curled with her feet up. 'Move those Adrian darling, will you? Sit down somewhere Dave. Adrian, see to the kettle, pet lamb?' Mum tweaks the crocheted blanket, as though modest, so that it reaches down her brown tights to fully cover her toes, while Dave clumsily tugs off his boots then pads towards an easy chair, keeping a respectful distance.

I don't remember Mum ever being well. She never gets anywhere with the doctors. They said the thing last Sunday was due to the stress of moving, not a serious attempt, and that I wasn't to worry. They increased her medication.

I go into the kitchen, put the kettle on, and hover, looking at the rain. I'm itching to get back to my room. Dave's visits are a nuisance, and embarrassing. He can't help her.

The clock, which is always a bit wrong, shows it's two-ish. I normally have a quick online chat with my friend Kaz around now. If I leave it much later, everyone's in bed in Japan. Kaz is my age and totally agrees with my opinions. Our favourite character is The Doctor, a hologram who's physically present, being a matter-light projection. His brain is a computer, a concept which I don't find too far-fetched. Online, we argue with other fans about the best uniform, the best characters, the best movie so far. The latter has to be *Star Trek II* in terms of plot and action: the one where Spock gets killed and is reincarnated. Kaz and I have this ongoing dispute with a bunch of Americans about practically everything. There's a guy aged seventy-four in Los Angeles, Ernesto, who we let join in cos he's cool, but the rest of us are between age thirteen (that's me) and twenty-two.

When I return from the kitchen with mugs and a fresh pot of tea, Dave has pulled some resources out of his bag: 'Fun with Maths at Key Stage Three' is the one on top.
'Adrian, my man!'
He tries too hard, does Dave.
'I'm just telling your mother: a teacher friend of ours managed to purloin a few useful resources from where she works. Especially maths stuff. It's so important isn't it, maths . . .' He trails off, seeing Mum's look.
I set down the tea tray. 'Thanks Dave. I'll have a look at them.'
Mum's little dry cough has been building up since Dave arrived. She keeps flapping her hand in front of her face as though a bit of air movement might help. 'No, no, I'll be alright,' she says bravely when I stand up, wanting to do something for her.
'It's been the dust,' she explains to Dave, getting right away from the subject of school books. 'I try to clean; keep on top of everything . . .'
'I must say you do marvellously well,' remarks Dave, looking round our spotless living room. 'You must get a lot of help from Adrian and Bob to keep it this tidy.'
'Actually, no.' I refute this, on the defensive. He suspects that I do housework instead of school work. 'Mum does the lot – she's a manic cleaner. Can't stop her once she gets going.'
Dave's eyebrows shoot up, looking at Mum flaked out on the couch.
'At night!' says Mum, annoyed. Then in a wan voice she says – 'sleep patterns,' by way of explanation. 'I don't sleep any more. Not like normal people. Soon as Bob comes upstairs I'm bright as a button. I've tried everything. My bio-rhythms are all out of sync. I end up cleaning the house all night, trying to tire myself out.'
'Actually I was hoping Bob would be about,' says Dave; 'I can offer him a bit of work repainting the chapel if he's available.'
As if he's not available.

Dave is looking around foolishly as though my Dad might be pottering behind the couch. Mum told me her illness makes Dave nervous. People can't cope with it. That's what makes it even harder. Vicious circle, she says, in her desperate voice, on one of those nights when she never stops hugging me, stroking my hair.

'Depends, really,' says Mum. 'If he earns, they just dock it off the benefits. Don't suppose you'll be offering cash in hand, with it being the chapel.'

Dave clears his throat, perched in an uncomfortable way on the edge of the armchair. 'Harrum. Er, we've missed Bob in the village since you came out here,' he continues.

That's Dave being patronising. Dad hardly said a word to anyone in four years.

'Missed you all, of course!' He gestures at me – 'Couldn't make it to Y.P.F. this time, then?'

I hold up my hands again, indicating my project: 'I've been busy.' I was hoping that our moving to the end of a track three miles up the dale would finally get me out of going to Young People's Fellowship. All they talk about is school: teachers, homework, exams; who snogged who on the field. And Dave's wife tries to draw me in, asking what I've been studying in my week.

'Actually there's something that I do want to talk about with you and I was hoping I could speak to you all. I mean, as a family,' says Dave, suddenly quite assertive.

'Shall I go look for Dad?' I ask Mum, moving towards the door. Mum has started one of her coughing fits, flapping her hand at me to wait. Dave looks embarrassed, doesn't know what to do, as though he'd started her off somehow. In her broken 'cough' voice she wheezes at me between hacks, 'Sweetheart – my inhaler.' In fact, it's my inhaler, according to the prescription on the side, from way back. Luckily for Mum, I've never ever needed it, as Mum needs it by her. I go and pick it up from the cabinet right next to her and put it into her hand. She does wheezy breathing for ages, lying back on the cushions with her eyes closed. We wait. Dave isn't used to it.

'She'll be alright,' I tell him.

Dave looks at me seriously. 'You've probably guessed it's about you being home-educated,' he says, darting a nervous glance at my reclining mother.

She's listening.

'I'll get Dad, shall I?' I ask Dave this time, and immediately scoot out of the door without waiting for an answer. I'll feel disloyal to Mum if I allow this conversation to begin. 'I think I know where he is,' I call from the passage before disappearing.

The cottage is structurally a mess, but cheap to rent. I shudder to think of how cold it'll be when winter comes, having no heating upstairs.

Colder than the council house, without a doubt. But that was one of Mum's reasons for us moving out: the central heating being bad for our asthma. There was also double-glazing, another health hazard apparently, in that it creates a sealed, unchanging atmosphere in which dust mites thrive, causing allergies.

Mum also hated the lack of privacy. People calling in, and then the inevitable gossip; people's opinions.

I hurry across the drizzly yard, feeling a bit agitated: time's ticking on. Kaz will give up on me and shut down before long.

Sure enough, Dad is where I expect him to be: sitting in our car in the dilapidated corrugated iron structure that serves as a garage, listening to his cassettes. We watch TV in the afternoons, Mum and I, whereas Dad comes out in all weathers to listen to his cassettes. Especially the last few days.

The garage is still piled up with crates to unpack, plus all Dad's junk – stuff that he makes things with. On top of one crate is our hi-fi which broke in the move, semi-dismantled. I squeeze between two opened boxes of machine components of some kind, sorted into metal and plastic. I take after my Dad – always tinkering.

'Dad!'

He's wearing headphones, sitting peacefully in the front seat, eyes closed. He makes people like Dave chuckle: the incongruity of a cassette-player and headphones installed in a Morris Minor. In the village he was famous for having a PhD; the eccentric scientist type.

'Dad,' I crank the door open, poke his arm, 'it's Dave.' Up close to Dad's bald head is pretty unpleasant: it's gone fiery red on top, encrusted with psoriasis. Beneath the struggle of hair that starts above his ears and dangles in curling, hippyish strands down his neck, the red and flaking skin continues until it reaches his denim jacket. It used to be only in patches. I can see the same colouration flooding out from under his sleeves, sneaking onto the backs of his hands.

Dad follows me indoors to be polite to Dave. He's quiet, but always pleasant, my Dad.

Mum has put a damper on Dave's suggestion about the school, about the scholarship, by starting to choke.

'Actually the Morris needs a bit of work,' my Dad is explaining in his gentle, apologetic way to Dave, declining his offer of work, while Mum carries on in the background. 'Can't get her down the track at the moment.'

Dave looks alarmed. 'You mean . . . you're all stuck here? What about shopping? Have you got what you need?'

Mum has that chalk-white complexion she gets when she hyperventilates. The choking usually sets her off on a panic-attack. I know she'll calm down when Dave leaves, so I pull him by the arm towards the passage. He's got enough sense to know when it's time to go.

Outside I accompany Dave slowly, kicking leaves all the way, to his tin-box Renault 2CV.

'You're looking a bit despondent,' says Dave, looking hard into my face. 'You didn't give your own opinion on the matter.'

'I'm not well enough,' I sigh, swamped by a wave of resignation. 'Anyway, neither is she. I can't leave her.'

'It's your Dad's job to look after your Mum,' says Dave. 'You're a clever lad,' he calls, folding himself into his car. 'You could do well.'

The little red car scuttles out of sight between the trees and I'm left with a screeching owl, then silence.

Mum is only able to sip water after Dave has left. I have to put a bucket near the couch for if she's sick. They don't know what to do about the choking. Apparently she's got a blockage that they can't find.

It's frustrating, having everything totally perfect in my Space Station except for a red cover for my bed, and no means of getting one. But then, there's no-one to show it to anyway. I've described it in great detail to Kaz, but the trouble with being online is, people are always telling you these amazing things they've done and you know they can get away with the biggest lies in the world.

I put my uniform on for my one-to-one with Kaz, who is still up at one a.m. Japanese time without his parents knowing. I tell him I'm often up until it gets light, as my parents never come up to check. I explain that we all stay up at night in my family, then sleep in until about midday.

I normally log on again at around ten in the evening, when the American kids are just home from school. Kaz, being in Japan, is the odd one out: he gets on to us as the night goes on, fitting in a half-hour when he first wakes up, before he goes off to college. In the States there's Jon, Mahmet and Gary, Lester and Ernesto, and a few more who are off and on.

Tonight the paint smell in my room has given me a headache. I only notice it properly when I log off. It's three in the morning. Mum stopped bumping around with the vacuum cleaner a while ago. At the last soft crackle of the monitor extinguishing itself I get that pang. If only Kaz lived in the village. If only the kids in the village were like Jon, Mahmet, Gary, and Lester.

I'm chilly. It's blacker inside my room than out: the curtainless window is a ghostly square hovering in a void. I grope for my lamp to see myself into bed, feeling like when you've just watched the best movie ever and suddenly it's over and you have to look round you and acknowledge the real world again.

I speculate that most U.S. boys are probably like my internet friends. I'm not negative enough to think that everyone of my age is like the Y.P.F. kids – brain-dead and into snogging each other. I pick up the prospectus Dave left, for one more look. The loose form for applying for a bursary slips to the floor. The smell of the glossy paper is like a stimulant. Poring over the photos, breathing it in, I get excited.

The square of my window has turned a pale yellow by the time I pull my quilt over my head. I imagine, out there, in the gloom, a group of boys like me, snoring away in a big dormitory. They're all interested in *Star Trek*, and science, and computers. We've each got a PC next to our beds, and every night, we mess about in our dormitory, doing homework, getting on the internet, having a go on each other's play stations.

I don't sleep well: the drone of the Morris engine becomes insistent. Dad always works on stuff through the night. By six thirty it's fully light outdoors. The trees throw their green shade into my room and I stare at my gold alarm clock, wondering what else would look good painted gold.

I decide to get up, open the window, let some more of the heavy paint smell disperse. My bedroom walls still feel tacky. My uniform is crumpled with bits of fluff stuck to the black fabric from being worn in bed.

It's as though the garage is alive, humming, like it's a giant machine. Nothing wrong with the Morris. It's been running for hours. Literally.

I turn abruptly from the window. The dark walls are suddenly caving in on me. I bolt for the landing, my brain zinging from the paint smell, the engine noise, the black silence behind it all. I pound down the stairs, then stop sharply: I should be as quiet as possible; creeping.

In the passage the vacuum cleaner is lying half out of the understairs cupboard. The hose is missing: only an inch of it pokes from the red body of the machine, the rest having been sliced off unevenly. The stanley knife is lying on the little table by the phone.

The sitting room door is slightly ajar. The electronic tones of the digits as I dial the number resound in the passage, terrifyingly loud. It takes ages and ages for someone to answer. Eventually a sleepy, enquiring male voice is in my ear.

'Dave,' I whisper, 'It's Adrian. Look, I've decided . . .' The Morris engine is running in my head – 'Look, I want to go to that school. Can you come and get me?'

'Uh?'

Dave isn't with it. '*Listen.*' My voice is rising.

Mum's drowsy murmur floats from the sitting room: 'Adrian?'

I burst out crying; I can't help it. 'Dave! Can you come and pick me up – *I want to go to that school.*'

Sylvia Goodman

Skilled Worker

He spends his days peering
Into cheerless caverns
Shining lamps into damp spaces.
Some may emanate sweetness
Others odours redolent of decay,
Neglected tombs of joyful times.
Ranged in the wet warm darkness
Rear up the standing rocks
Deep-rooted white in rose-hued beds.
Some crags discoloured
Cracked and fissured
Teeter in amaranthine gloom.
His silvery instruments
Flash and glint reflecting
Movement of his twisting wrist.
He probes the noisome depths
Casts jets of water, blasts of air.
An adamantine surface
Pierced, a bridge in place,
A brace applied. He toils
Unchallenged among cavities.
His wordless victim lies
Supine and tense, fists clenched
The whole world contracted
To a white coat, a whining drill.

Plea

A wheeling snowstorm feathers round my head
The east wind bites and scores my tearful face
My heart is ice recalling what you said
And home has ceased to be a hallowed place.
The air is sharp, the ground is white with frost
Your words keep whirling wildly in my brain
Before you spoke did you not count the cost
To us, to them, to all who'll bear the pain?
Perhaps the frozen night had chilled your heart
And when the sun shines warm your wrath will melt
You'll think again, repine your unkind part
Regret the harshness of the blow you dealt.
   I beg you, darling, let your anger go
   Lest I submerge and drown in anguished woe.

Sylvia Goodman

Fragile Memories

Have you forgotten me? I still dream
Of days we spent in heedless bliss.
When your youthful memories teem
Am I wrapped in your happiness?

Do you remember me, or did I fade
Within the year, a month or two?
Am I wrong, or had you strayed
So soon in search of someone new?

Did you discard me? I despaired
Yet hope held fast, a steely halter.
In all my dreams and prayers you cared
For how I loved you!

                              Time can't alter
Memories of kisses taken, given
Walks in moonlight by the river.
Sun-blessed caresses I can summon.

All such memories make me shiver.

For now I wonder, do I dream?
And was our youth a joyful time?
Or was there deep inside a scream
Because we sought a paradigm

Of what young love should really be
From films we'd seen and books we'd read
Yet quite remote from you and me.

Deny these thoughts! I'm filled with dread.

My love to you was fierce and strong.
Could memory lie? I recall pain
And tear-soaked pillows all night long.

Did we once linger down a lane?
Was this our real past together –
Our phone calls all the life we shared?

Was this the love I thought a tether?
Yet still my heart's forever snared.

Sylvia Goodman

African Statue

Why does he cry so loud?
He is not of my world.
Is he homesick
Living among such gentle greenery?
Is the light too misted for him
Leaving him stifled?
He whose horizon lies thirty miles away
Where he can reach out
To touch the nomad camels
As they disappear.
Is the autumn sky
Too fragrant with rain?
He opens his mouth so wide.
Is it to catch the sacred drops
So anxiously awaited in his country,
So shruggingly dismissed in mine –
"Another nasty day"?
Or does he gasp for breath
Desperate for the desert air
Sullied by sand,
But unpolluted by our raucous fumes.
I am not of his world.
The desert camels and the sand
Are not for me.
Yet I am uneasy in his presence
I fear him and his elemental needs.
I have lost his joy in the rain
And the crispness of the clear October light.
The city's rush and rumble overwhelm
And heedless I inhale its exhalations.
I am too much of our world
And he recalls me constantly to his.

Sylvia Goodman

Bad Weather Coming

A swirl of grey sweeps up the sky
The sun too soon renounces day
As human traffic hurries by
Intent on leaving work for play.

The sun too soon renounces day
Denying light and warmth to us
Intent on leaving work for play
Who now must queue to catch a bus.

Denying light and warmth to us
Means colds and flu could soon arrive.
Who now must queue to catch a bus?
The ones least able to survive.

Mean colds and flu could soon arrive
To give us coughs and make us sneeze
The ones least able to survive
Could well expire with gasp or wheeze.

To give us coughs and make us sneeze
The winter's cold and wet conspire
And soon the old with gasp or wheeze
Could enter in the heavenly choir.

The winter's cold and wet conspire
To smite the old, and babes in arms
Could enter in the heavenly choir
Too soon reduced to singing psalms.

They smite the old and babes in arms
As human traffic hurries by.
Too soon reduced to singing psalms
They swirl in grey, sweep up the sky.

Sean Burn

hard walkin yr old mans shadow

jazz, like sex, was illicit back then. we fucked without condoms stealin money to buy tapes of coltrane, miles, monk, carla ... bley, others, i dont recall 1/2 the names of drummers but i remember their patterns; their rhythms, a shot of caffeine buzzin ma arms, ma head, adrenalin pumpin, good as the best lay i ever had. poundin. animalistic. goin ballistic, prayin his daa would never catch us. if music be the food of love, rut on.

ma own was different, he treated us fair, his wean, cradled safe in rockin chair, rock-a-bye-babby back & forth long as i wanted, wakin after ma appendix burst to find him teary eyed, strokin us with those warm worn hands, our 1st gig, him standin, clappin, wouldnt stop; aye, his hands was magic

he made strings weep; pulled tears from cor anglais, & coaxed the clownin trombones to sing. those hands led the greatest of orchestras, tugged the heartstrings of europe. they even flew him to the states, travel had an edge back then, before i was bom. flyin, an accolade, he soared like icarus. & fell like him too. stormy times. with orchestras, with lovers, male & female, with public & press, many said bastard to his face, but to us he was always daa; encouragin us to spread ma wings, we kept a parrot for years, folks called it cruel, daa called him oskar. that bird flew where it wanted, shat everywhere, daa knew how our brazilian grey felt, mind wantin to soar; hands & arms & wrists bound to earth.

was always tappin, i couldnt stop. drove ma folks nuts before they split, used to tap all the time. mealtimes. on the bus. lamp posts, gates, walls, tap tap tap tappity tap a 1 a 2 a 1 2 3, shuffle shuffle, tap tap tap a cra-a-ash, wap, wallop, bap-bap, tickety tickety tap. thats us. nerves or somethin. like bitin nails, this guy was sent to find out what was wrong, we just talked about sounds & stuff, us drummin on the desk, him batterin back. call & response, he was real cool, gave us a pair of sticks, said to take it out with 'em.

lord, i hated school orchestras, all that practisin when others was out footballin or fightin or chasin boys, girls, boys. 1 teacher, wee speccy git 4 foot nothin, used to bring in this home made podium for conductin. we was workin hard towards another bloody concert, givin music a bad name so we'd hate it enough to inflict on the next generation, anyhow, his stagin gives way, collarbone smashes, we give round of applause, no 1 workin out i loosened some screws, hammered out the wood. learnin to fight for what i believed, music became an obsession & a freedom & mostly a way of stickin 2 fingers up, like watchin daa do *faust*, & i mean do. shriekin. tempestous. violent cantata from russia with lust. daa loved new music, playin the hardest scores; gobblin em up like they was nothin. *faust*! a desperate howlin passion, clingin to life, crescendin thru anarchy, all 'em suits shocked like i was fistin lovers arse.

ma 1st album, durin punk mind, was porgy & bess. miles davis. gil evans. gershwin. cool. real cool. *prayer*, an answer to all of mine. i'd hit ma desk ma chair ma lamp ma bed wearin sticks out all the time splintered smashed trashed carashed. all those panes of glass headbutted, cars too close gettin kicked, stoved in. it wasnt wild, just workin it all out, findin the right channel, used all ma cash buyin more sticks savin up for ma own drumkit, wantin to be elvin jones stormin this tight wee club. his sweat hittin us full on, beads of flung mercury, salt fightin to overcome the beer. max roach – the hardest bopper of all, thats what they said. & the indestructible art blakey cookin up violence in his psycho-kitchen. i worshipped at altar their unholy trinity, their rhythm coursin ma veins, their pulse ma heartbeat, everythin makin sense, drummin was passion & politics, sex. sexuality, fuckin. depression. exultation, it was life. it was ma blood.

what really hooked us was that cage of metal, don cherrys '86 gig. was addicted to 'em sounds evolvin in clusters of heat & noise, matter & anti-matter sent out with the bigbang. this guy in his reinforced percussion cage; generatin sound from everythin. all surface was drum to him; no longer instrument but headstate of warped ecstasy & cherrys toy trumpet playin games against that! genius, thats why jazz.

i admired me old man, but wanted to walk ma own path. theres no enough chaos in classics, tho he brought out the wildness, life imitatin art. sometimes its hard walkin yr old mans shadow, tho he always gave praise, *dont be ashamed son. live it. breathe it. believe it.* it was music for the both of us – his on the page, mine in ma head.

goin to tchaikovskys *pathetique*. that 3rd movement, a riot of fireworks explodin across the deepenin sky, til those final few moments – a quiet fadin. that long drawn out chord . . . to nothingness, hall was silent, stunned, we all knew it was his last concert, i couldnt concentrate, just wantin him offstage, no dragged down, arms achin like the crucifixion, i could feel his hands shakin, the nails hammerin his wrists, he was good man, but the depression, & the cripplin arthritis, they say both runs in families, hope to god i never end like that. his hands was his life & by then they lay twisted, misshapen, grotesque on his knees & him sittin in semi-darkness starin at those lumps of bone, weepin. the blueroom of depression got him & .... & then i was truly alone.

we got big gigs thru the summer, us wantin beyond the grave with requiem he would be proud of. drummin up a storm & playin to his memory at festivals across the south of france. pernod by the glass – tall, cool & cracked, grit of anise on tongues, dust wipped off pavements, us blowin em away outdoors. 2,000 punters. cooped close. pissed, bayin for blood, so i gave 'em it. by the pint. takin their glasses to pour over ma head, grindin the glass into ma skull, beer & blood pourin down & i'm lickin ma own salt, enjoyin it. pulse weakenin a bit now tho you couldnt tell from the rhythm of ma beat. reckon i must of lost too much. that, & the drink & the sweat, & the heat & the grief of memory, was rushed to casualty, but the reviews! i reckon was worth it.

    i'm recoverin now, learnin it all over again. 1st steps, basics, a steady pulse. tappin it out in 12/8. the fancy stuff will come. aye it will. theres no heaven, we make our own reality, but i reckon the old bastards smilin. & i'm gonna smile too.

David Swann

Boggarts

Bad Men roamed our town's edges:
back alleys, quarries, the wind-blown moors,

places they were trapped in when we left
for my uncle's farm, from which they glowered

as our car took us to a countryside
of older monsters – creatures who'd sulked

the long centuries, moaned with heifers
in the muck and straw of their Holes:

woolsacks with flaming eyes, who loathed
the quick: running water, laughter.

Who watched while you worked alone
close to the oaks by the soft-spot,

sowing troughs, tying gates with twine,
where water slowed, where bullocks called . . .

. . . places your fingers stalled, from which you ran
through fading light for the ford,

for that line on the edge of their world
which they could not cross,

which you splashed to the farm's hearth,
that drowsers' place – safe . . .

until dark, until some call from the night
woke you in fields around your bed –

the house a speck on the hill's shoulder
foam swirling in the room's corner –

and creatures that knew no borders
wading now through water on the dream's edge,

kicking stones in rage,
grinding their teeth like boulders.

David Swann
Pleasure

The kind old lady who ran the B&B
near the jail was telling me about her war:

how, as a clippie, she travelled London
on double-deckers. "It was like a dream,"

she said. "Like being free. Imagine it –
me, giving the whole wide world their tickets!"

Later, kids and the smallest county changed things,
but the city streets still led to her door.

She remembered the lodger she offered
a key to. It was his first night outside,

and he turned down the chance. "Her Majesty's
open prisons _give_ you keys," he explained,

"but I missed this thing they won't allow:
to dance up someone's step and press the bell."

A few pints on, he smiled when she answered
his ring: "Sometimes the small things are enough."

Later, on the same bed where the freed man
must have laid, I drift through Rutland's sleep:

empty streets and wind in summer trees,
birds singing to a lake, and the guitarist

trying to crack some old Black Sabbath dirge.
Tomorrow – a job interview, and change,

but, for now, give me these rough old chords
and an open window. Small things. Enough.

David Swann

Ghost train

Digging on an allotment, I think of tunnels,
and one leads me to the ghost train in Blackpool,
where our faces were flicked by plastic bats

and those screams returned in another tunnel:
the dark room of a cheap boarding house
where only my mother's touch of the switch

brought me back to the light . . . just as the sun
glinting on a spade restores the allotment,
where I have dug all morning into the tunnel

that runs through this poem, which leads beyond
the pleasure beach and climbs to the screams
of banged-up men in the prison I taught in,

where a con once told me he'd found a sea-shell
in the yard. *They say it's just noise in your head*,
he shrugged, and looked at his feet, as if hope

tapered out at the limit of his toes.
But that day when he found the shell and held
it to his ear, he walked its bright tunnel

and came out by the water – until lights-out
brought him back to the black soil of his cell
where he had spent years, digging, digging.

The angel of old men's shins

He says the jail's walls are the colour
of old drizzle and that everything in here
tastes like the early stages of 'flu,
smells of baggy ankle socks that perverts wear.

It doesn't matter. A guardian spirit
watches over him, and has been his calm
since he first put his stuff in the box
and she whispered he was safe from harm.

David Swann

He's not alone. The landings are roamed
by angels, who search out blokes
afraid of going under, the ones
that can't get out of their heads

or who have gone out of their heads
staring into the yard, whose eyes
have stalled in the sterile zone,
where nothing moves, only orange peels

against a fence, in the breeze.
Minor angels on the wind's breath:
guardians of watered gravy, shiny carpets,
old men's shins and metered tellies.

Our Lady Of The Scratchy Curtain Runners,
of the boarding house with thin black stairs.
Angel that steams from you at first light,
from the cold bed. Who falters, slips.

It doesn't matter. When wind comes
and blows petals against the wall,
he'll keep the faith. Stare into a drift
of white flowers, thankful that he's safe.

In the grotto

NO, the Lady Mayoress would NOT sit down!
"Mr Chairman – if we aren't careful,
these plans will turn that estate into a grotto."

It was the same speaker who'd once famously said,
"Mr Chairman, I would like to ask a remark",
which maybe explained the reaction in the chamber:

my fellow hacks fluttering coughs like writs,
expressing new interest in their biros and shins
and the precise location of emergency exits.

In the end, I lost count of the hours I spent
on speakers who said "at this time in point"
and demanded they be quoted word for word

David Swann

or the speeches I reported by the bloke
who felt the arts burned enough of our cash
"when we already have two brass bands each year."

I suppose they tried their best – harder, for sure,
than the press. We tended just to shake our heads
when trees were described as potential litter hazards

and drift, instead, to the council's empire
of terminuses and sheds, imagining gangs
of elves awaiting the word of the Lady Mayoress

to hit the streets and hustle snow, push gifts
on toddlers as young as five, and joy-ride
reindeers over the roofs of the grotto.

Noreen Rees

Jesus on a Nan Bread

Picture the church. For the moment it is empty, its ancient walls covered in a rash of mildew. A smell of damp timber hangs with the vestments in the choir cupboard, where old ledgers are jammed next to a cardboard box of rusting mouse traps. Sunlight filters through the stained glass windows, casting green and blue lozenges onto the scuffed wooden floor of the nave. Fragments of flaking ceiling are scattered like dandruff on the rood screen and, reaching up to the greying sky outside, is the belltower. Inside the church there is a silence so thick it could be sliced and bottled. But out in the car park two noises; a rock music CD being played loudly in a rusty Ford Fiesta, and a Renault Clio being driven at speed through the car park gates.

Arnold is late for church opening duty. Hasn't even had time for a slice of breakfast toast. And his parking space has been taken by a rusted Ford Fiesta with a mismatched door. Inside the car a young man is sitting at the wheel. He is listening to a loud music CD, and shaking his shaven head.

Arnold gets out of his car and adjusts his tie slightly. The young man is looking away and doing no harm, he supposes and anyway, Mrs Ellis and the other ladies of the church will be coming soon to finish off the Harvest flower arrangements. He won't be alone for long. The young man should be gone by then, and Arnold might have a chance to eat a snack while he waits for the visitors. He steps up to the church doorway, and begins to unlock the door. Inside the church (where the rain has come in regularly since the sixties) the walls are blotched like excema. Arnold wipes his polished shoes on the doormat. His footsteps echo in the empty space as he walks towards the light switch and flicks it on. He picks out the junk mail from the letter cage on the back of the door. Fortunately no spent fireworks as happened last year. There is an electricity bill, which he posts through the office door right at the back of the church. He looks at his watch. He should have put the notice board out ten minutes ago and opened for business as it were. But as he picks up the board the outside door opens and the young man from the Ford Fiesta comes in. Arnold's hands clench and he holds the board like a protective shield. Headlines he has read in the Daily Telegraph come into his mind. *Vicar mugged for fifty pence. Verger's church ordeal. Church worker found dead in graveyard.* But, the young man is wearing a clean jacket, and his T shirt has been pressed even though it reads "**** YOU."

The young man looks around him, blinking in the dull light. Then he asks "Are you the vicar?"

His voice is surprisingly soft. Arnold unclenches his hands, and puts the noticeboard down. He holds one hand out, then withdraws it self-consciously.

"Sorry. Father Blenkinsop is the vicar. Do you need him? Has someone died?"

"Oh, no."

"Well you can speak to me if you wish. It's my church duty today. I'm Mr Fowles." Arnold moves to a pew, pulls the knees of his cavalry twill trousers. "Sit down."

The young man sits, perched forward like a rook on a fence. There is an uneasy silence.

"What's your name?"

"David."

"Would you like me to pray with you, David?" The young man looks alarmed.

"Would you like to talk then ?" Arnold asks. He tries to sound sympathetic but really he hates this bit the most. Stealing, adultery, relationship breakdown. He's heard it all. Sometimes he feels as if people have taken the ten commandments and used them as a checklist for doing the opposite. He waits patiently for David to begin. There will be a catalogue of sins. There always is. Arnold's gaze rests on the Harvest fruit laid out on the communion rail. The apples and oranges gleam like traffic lights, and the smell seems to fill the church. He begins to feel slightly nauseous. He should have made time for breakfast.

"I wanted to show you this," David says at last.

Arnold focuses his eyes on the dahlias in the display above David's head. A feeling of dread descends upon him. What if it is something obscene? A symbol of the occult? A knife? The headlines swim before Arnold's eyes once more but when he looks down he is relieved to see David unwrapping what looks at first glance like a sandwich. The young man flips over the paper napkin to expose – what is it exactly?

"I went out for a curry last night," says David.

"Yes?"

"Well, this nan bread. It just looked normal, nothing wrong at all, but when I looked again. See."

Arnold squints in the inadequate lighting.

"It's Jesus."

"Beg pardon?"

"Jesus. There on my nan bread."

Arnold looks up to the plaque above the lectern. He often finds himself looking at it on church duty days. LORD GIVE ME STRENGTH it reads.

"Do you think it's a sign?" the young man asks.

Arnold recalls his church duty training. Listen and support. He takes out his glasses, puts them on, examines the nan bread, clears his throat loudly. "A sign?"

"Maybe – I don't know exactly. That's why I brought it here."

"Oh." Arnold looks at his watch. He has only been here fifteen minutes, and now his stomach is cramping and he is beginning to feel light-headed. Perhaps if he can get rid of David, he can pop over the road to the sandwich shop before the next visitor arrives. *Look interested. Give him five minutes then guide him to the door.*

"So you think it's become a sort of relic?" Arnold says.

"Yeah, that's what I mean."

"Hmm interesting," Arnold says, thinking exactly the opposite.

"Yes I can see some resemblance."

"So what will you do with it?" David slouches in the pew, legs splayed.

"Well, I could mention it to Father Blenkinsop. He will know what to do." Arnold looks at his watch. Still an hour's duty to go. He can feel the blood rushing round his head, making him dizzy. This is clearly going to be a long haul. He feels a sharp pain in his empty stomach. Still no Mrs Ellis. David might not be quite as keen to tell his story if her gargoyle face is peering down at them while polishing the altar cross.

"And there's something else."

Arnold could have guessed it. David produces a lighter from inside his leather jacket.

"Mind if I smoke?"

"I'm sorry. It's not allowed. Fire regulations," Arnold explains. Has David been in a fight? Had an affair? Is he on drugs? David puts away his cigarettes and leans forward.

"I've got a bairn that needs seeing to, christening or whatever. So what do I have to do?"

Arnold feels his heart slow. "Are you married?"

"No, but it's mine. I had the DNA test."

Arnold sighs. "Your baby's mother. Do you – er – live with her?"

"No way . . . But I do want my bairn done." David takes out a photograph of a sleepy child. She is wearing a miniature football shirt and hat.

"That's Kylie. What a belter eh?"

"Yes," says Arnold. "Very unusual."

"I want things to be done properly. For her."

Arnold's eye flicks to the names on the cradle roll. Seventy years ago his name was added, in black calligraphy. In those days every child had their name put down. Or almost every. But there were some in his school class who were never allowed to attend the outings and parties. Those excluded because of their parents, or lack of . . . Arnold feels a sense of shame. What became of those children, the outcasts? He takes out his fountain pen and writes a note.

"Here is Father Blenkinsop's number. You'll need to talk to him about a christening, if you're sure that's what you want."

"Oh right, I do."

Arnold begins to get up. But the pew seems to be sliding beneath him. The aisle is telescoping away. If only he'd eaten breakfast.

"Are you alright mate?"

David's voice is far away, behind what sounds like a waterfall. When Arnold comes to, he is stretched out in one of the pews.

"You had me going there, mate. Thought you were a gonner."

Arnold's hand reaches up to his neck. His tie has been undone.

"Did a first aid course ages ago," says David in explanation. "Hope you didn't mind me loosening your clothes. I honestly thought you'd had it."

"I feel much better now thanks. Do you think you could get me a drink of water? There's a sink behind the door over there." David moves away and Arnold begins to sit up slowly. His head still feels like a washing machine on a fast spin cycle. A thought strikes him. He shoots his hand to his inside jacket pocket making sure David is not looking. Yes, his wallet is still there. Quickly he looks inside. Nothing missing. He feels ashamed for the second time that morning.

The young man is coming up the aisle towards him, spilling water from what looks like a flower vase. "Couldn't find no cups, sorry."

Arnold drinks gratefully, ignoring the green algae round the rim and the woody smell of cut stems.

"Well, best be off then." David pats his shirt pocket. "I'll be in touch with Mr Blenkinsop about Kylie. You'll be O.K. won't you?"

"Oh, yes. Mrs Ellis and her flower ladies will be here soon."

"So, I'll leave this here then shall I?" David thrusts the nan bread into Arnold's hand. He can feel the rough paper napkin, smell the baked dough beneath.

"See you then, mate." David's leather jacket creaks as he opens the outside door. The door clangs shut.

Arnold puts the water jar down, and ponders the choice of sandwiches that will be available at the shop. Coronation chicken? Roast beef with horseradish? Maybe bacon and tomato sausage? He almost runs to the outside door.

But he can see the deadlock lying across the chink of light. He feels for the keys in his pocket. He had them when he came in. Where has he put them? Then he realises he has probably posted them through the office door with the electricity bill. There is a brush draught excluder on the bottom of the office door. There is no way of pushing anything through to retrieve the keys. Arnold is locked inside the church. And his last meal was fourteen hours ago.

And where is Mrs Ellis? He hopes she hasn't tripped on the old lino tiles in her scullery at home, is lying sprawled on the floor, unable to reach her phone. Arnold thinks of the sandwich shop – of saveloys and pease pudding, chicken and stuffing, ham and salad. All unavailable. All outside the locked door.

He returns to the pew and takes another sip of water. There is a hint of turpentine in it. Perhaps Mr Lewis the caretaker has used it to wash his brushes in. Arnold feels sick and shaky now. He tries the office door on the off chance that it isn't locked, then the other door which leads through to the vestry. All locked. He makes his way back to the pew and sits down. After eleven. Mrs Ellis is at least half an hour late. And where are the other ladies? They've always been here on other church duty days.

He listens for the sound of a key in the lock. There is nothing. Only the faint scraping of a twig across the window, the soft moaning of the wind in the belltower. Arnold can hear a rushing in his ears, like sand being slapped by the sea. He has got the right day hasn't he? They will be here soon? He doesn't want to be alone much longer. He might start to think about things, about the past, about Jessie. How he misses her.

His fingers touch the wrapped nan bread in his pocket. He pulls it out and opens it. There is clearly something there – a dribble of curry sauce perhaps, a shaking of turmeric. Is it a trick of the light? Remarkable, but it does seem to resemble the face of Jesus. The face of Jesus as painted by El Greco perhaps.

He takes another sip of turpentine-water and rubs the bread with his finger. A small piece has broken off. It smells of yeast and spices. He puts it to his mouth.

Several minutes later, Mrs Ellis opens the door. The church opener is slumped in the pew. His suit is dishevelled and covered in crumbs and he is muttering something about eating Jesus. "Eating Jesus indeed," Mrs Ellis says taking out her mobile phone from her handbag and ringing for an ambulance. "You need a good woman to look after you, that's all. Need a bit of feeding up, regular meals." The church opener closes his eyes. There is no sound except for the steady buffing noise of cloth on brass and the faint sound of an ambulance siren coming nearer.

Jacqui Rowe

Before the Funeral

It's a nuisance that Barbara had to die
when my legs are all aching from walking round town
and none of the shops with so much as a chair
any more. The Independent Grocers and those WI
women are bound to be there, looking down
their noses, singing Jerusalem, as if you're not there.

I suppose I'll have to wear the suit I got for their
Golden Wedding again because I'll die
if I have another disaster in town
looking for shops that have gone, and a chair.
My legs can't cope with the strain. I
keep telling that osteopath, it gets me down.

She gives me little pills from France. Down
by where that Barbara used to live, they're
beginning to dig up the pavement. She'd die.
well, of course she already has. In town,
just before Leonard phoned – I needed a chair,
I was so shocked when I heard; I

always thought he'd be the first – anyway, I
saw a really nice jacket in Marks, down
from forty five pounds, in navy. There
was nothing wrong with it but I'd have to dye
my shoes and I can't face going to town
again. I'll end up in a wheelchair,

the way I'm going. I might get a chair
lift; the stairs make my legs ache and my one eye
goes blurred when I try to look down
in these new glasses. I don't know why they're
still not right. Every week someone seems to die
and the funeral's always in the middle of town –

I suppose there's more room in that church in town –
Leonard's asked so many. There'll hardly be a chair,
what with all the hangers on, by the time I
get there. Afterwards, they'll be shovelling down
some dried up sandwiches. A free meal's all they're
going for. Just like that Barbara to have to die

now, when town's so crowded. If I were to die
no one would know for hours. I could go now, in this chair.
That condolence card's there. I'll just write my sympathy down.

Jacqui Rowe

Unexposed

You were never in there,
        one leg paperclip bent
    up to your shoulder,
  the Printemps carrier a decoration on your chest.
Beneath the blue checked brim
      you watched the line towards Auvers,
        unimpressed upon emulsion,
        altering no dyes,
        chemically unchanged amongst the silver salts.
Like Sacre Coeur,
like Oscar Wilde's sarcophagus,
like effigies across the Seine,
            your rays never passed into the chamber
             you were not made transparent
                or glossed or trimmed.
    I do not keep you under glass
              but here
              in this.

Poisoning the Garden

Poisoning the garden, I think of my father
who said, "They wouldn't call it work
if it wasn't," pumping the acid
smelling heat from the casting shop
into his arteries. He gave away
his hearing to the coining press, sold
his soul to the rolling mill.
When they used the Morris Oxford
because we had no phone, he nursed
the boiler while the daytime men
drank, on Saturdays talked down holes,
leading a child through the glamour
of oil and copper blanks.

Each year, as the dahlias showed,
he broke up, brittle, looking for a point
down Dorset lanes. Six honest serving men
supporting him through stamps and into fuchsias.
Half standard *Thalia* and *Mrs Lovell-Swisher*
went for lower than a third, though
he put his heart into the greenhouse
he bricked and glazed around them.

Jacqui Rowe

She Means Distant Lies

Shameless, nameless,
    he detests distress,
        blames the best, beats the rest.
  She means distant lies,
  tries the East as dharma, Brahma
is a shaman then a lama.
He, as marble, snarls at balm,
    hears alarms,
      stares at maids in shades that stain,
        meets her train.
Mild as mist she smiles,
    dials.
      Later, brainless, aimless
        stabs his harmless tears
          and sneers.
            He leers,
    has been seen in better states,
retains the strains,
    he estimates.
  In satin dresses, she learns Latin,
      earns a mint,
        hints at trends,
          bends, lends.
Mirthless, earthless,
    he dismantles her maternal heart,
binds internal and eternal tides,
    abides in meatless shambles,
            eats.
    In a barn she hesitates, meditates.
      Intimates send darts; it starts.
  Miasma, asthma, tired straits and debt destabilise,
disable air
  in Eire and Tibet,
      blend nine times ten
      times three times
        mine times thine,
            mend ire and he and she,
      astern, a star at sea.
        As barmen, airmen, starmen steer,
          near brine in lanes, slime in rain,
lead them there.
  Battle metal
  rattle mantra and mandala,

                      blast the tabla, master streams.
Dreams, mental arias, elate.
          Their stale debate sails blatant in the drains
                    In sterile bile,
                                  slides, denies, elides, dies

Seeing Puppies in the Dark

I
This is the dark time of the year
when a black dog could disappear,
                            reappear,
                  swallow fear,
                      be near.

II
Then Eva she put the toe of her slipper
underneath Rags and the broken haired terrier,
the little one and she shifted them off the hearth.
And the old man, my father, he come home
and he says, "Whose blinking Dalmatian is this?"
You're more a setter than a pointer, you.
He took old Rags away and he brought him back
and from that day he left the sheep alone.
What did he do? the old woman always asked.
We never knew,

III
What did the Gordons know,
            leaping
                      from torn paper to fill
     the dog shaped hole
                              in your aura?

IV
                                    We pass the cold line at 5
                        where the magpie leaves
                                the clear picked leg bone
                                            from a tabby cat.
I have left the photograph I took
but did not take: On Site Ebony 1992 to 1993

V
NAMES FOR A PUPPY,
BECAUSE HE IS A DOG: Sirius

BECAUSE HE MAY BE BLACK: Ebony Shadow Jet
BECAUSE HE IS GERMAN: Rolf Kaspar Axel Klaus
BECAUSE HE IS A GERMAN HUNTER: Jaeger Nimrod
BECAUSE HE WILL COME TO US AT CHRISTMASTIME:
   Noel Yul Santa's Little Helper Robin
BECAUSE IT MAY BE BOXING DAY: Vacslav
BECAUSE HE WAS BORN ON AGINCOURT DAY: Henry Crispin
   Zeb
AFTER HIS FATHER AND MY CHILD UNCLE: Abel

VI
In a strip of what my grandmother called the scullery
              all I see is my mother's wide collared
red coat
       and her shoulders weeping or as I would say crying
                                 which adults did
                for the deaths of uncles I had never seen
     because they lived in rooms. She mourns the promise of a house
              and I know there will not be a dog.

VII
       By the Peter Pan statue
          you asked me about the spaniel who stayed
close while the other
          ran around us
                  on the Midsummer day before
                         my thirteenth birthday
and I cried
                because it was my happiest day
        before I had you.

VIII
Four Quartets weather.
     It would be ten thirty on a July evening
     and we sing,
        "We wish o little kissing Santa Claus"
         at minus nought point five
      the sunset blushing broad leaves clinging alive on branches
dark as late as five o'clock
here in the south a week before the shortest day.

IX
In the dark time of the year
he vanished in the moon's eclipse.

Jacqui Rowe

Munsterländers never go;
you find them by their white tail tips.

X

                                      Because my mother taught me to doubt
                                          I walked around, to both of you,
                                              the truth of which I wanted,
expecting that, by saying,
                the dark one would be taken when we got there
            leaving the half-tailed,
                          lightest one we probably would have
                                  loved as much.

Jay Merill

TimeShare

Those who have bought into the Timeshare will sit by a Hockneyesque blue pool with smoky-iced drinks in chunky glasses, they will be invited to a party later and dance at the most fantastic disco in the world. Because they've made it, have passed the test, they will experience the sensation of a sweet relief, shriven at last of any further responsibility. Coming down to now, landing, it's all o'kay and they needn't go through the agony of it again. A pool of chemical blue, shaped traditionally like a kidney or a bean, a line of Californian palm trees shutting out sight of the fence, a taut fringed sunshade informing them that they are in a tropical location. Waitresses done out like holidaycamp hostesses with plastic lilies in their hair and goldspray face paint, pose by the pool awaiting orders. They swivel their bodies half round the tables when they're serving, making dancing motions with their feet.

All of this. The buyers drink through straws like rewarded children, happy to believe in their own discovered goodness, to have pulled through, made it to the better side of life. They are relieved politely, for the sake of everybody involved, smile in bewilderment at the one or two other couples still sitting at their tables. All in it together sort of look, *for better or worse*, a wedded feel; and a not quite knowing whether they are foolish or should be proud. Beyond the pool a line of clear cut little yellow chalets. Yellow for south, for sun, setting off the pool's unnatural, paintbox blue. They sip the sweetish alcoholic drinks, reminding themselves that it's really happening, they are undeniably here. This is the life they'll have here from now on, in the annual two weeks they own the place – a dream which they have already agreed to pay for. Except to them in this enchanted moment the whole thing has the quality of the eternal about it, nobody's thinking about the length of time. And they can be let alone now, start to look at the thing as an achievement, part of the new-look them, a choice they have successfully made.

All this is what Melita is reflecting upon as she takes in the sight of the pool and chalets, the scattered tables on sparse thin bladed grass. Glow of their glasses with the golden liquid, chunklets of ice which click when you swirl, such a good noise that. And Melita tries to visualise the dimensions of it all, tries to tap into the meaning, sum it up for herself, because at first she couldn't quite see what exactly was going on here.

The colours, smells and concepts are just slightly dated models of perfection, but maybe people buy because underneath the idea of glamour it's really a comfort thing they're opting for, a compromise situation, something known and homey on the underside. Or maybe it's the only *glamour* they can afford. Of course Melita had stepped back

Jay Merill

from purchasing her bit of the dream, hadn't been one of those who'd said *I will*. She and Leo were not, as a consequence, invited to the party but were hastily said goodbye to at the door. Unceremonious, yet there had been a flavour of ritual about the way the door was held wide open for them with a dismissive hand. And at the same moment she had seen the welcomed received figures of the other couples, the *good* ones with their clearcut relief already starting to drown out the embarrassment of first realisation. They are already getting used to the idea they've bought, the shock of it is waning and they're preparing to enjoy this comfortable semi-detached holiday dream which Melita could not in the end believe in. You're either *one of us* or you're out of it. Melita's out, and so is Leo by association. Does he mind that, it's hard to say. They're through the door in secs, already on the road, an alarmingly quick transition here from the glitzy floorshow to the street beyond the fence. The same sun out there but how drab it seems by comparison, suddenly. Melita half wishes she was enclosed again, sitting under a striped umbrella on the crazy paved terrace eating salted peanuts and small orange coloured crunchy things tasting vaguely of cheese. A chosen one. She glances at Leo but it's never easy to read what he's thinking. She'd thought earlier he'd looked reproachful when she'd resisted the hard sell, as though he'd have preferred her to give in gracefully.

But it's hard to say for sure. Not that Leo would have liked the two of them to come here on a regular basis. The last thing, surely, he would have wanted. But as they walk down the darkening road he doesn't look altogether happy. He seems a bit distant, kicks at a few loose pebbles with the toe of his running shoes. She even wonders whether he wants the *two of them* at all or whether he'd rather hang onto being just the one. There'd be no point in asking him either. It would sound too negative and anyway he's not so good at giving the straight answer. Another year has passed since that glimpse into the world of *TimeShare*. Melita still doesn't quite know what's happening with Leo. Sometimes he acts so close to her that it's a shock when he withdraws himself, acts cool, seems to disappear from her life for whole chunks of time. He's away working of course, but she doesn't mean that. It's an emotional withdrawal she senses, as though being close to someone is too intense a thing to be experienced undiluted and he can't carry on with it for very long. There have to be gaps.

Waiting at the street sign and here comes Leo in wicked black clothes, wearing no other colour, as though he won't try and confuse you by making ambiguous statements. Wearing shiny black, even the shirt, even the buttons on the shirt, everything. How does she bear with this over concentration of his on the colours he's wearing, today wanting only the one, sometimes wanting a mish-mash of as many colours as possible, but either way never forgetful. He's always making a statement of some kind stylistically, but does it have any value, she can't help asking herself. It's usually the case that Melita judges him harshly the first time she's seeing him after ages. She's easily irritated by the look of him, and also she wonders how much is the result of a build up of resentment at his absence. But very quickly she relents and then forgets. Leo has placatory qualities that help things blow over before you'd believe it possible. In no time at all here she'll be, making excuses for him, or not noticing the annoying traits.

Curious that hold he has over Melita despite everything. She'll never stand out against Leo for very long even though in theory, when he isn't there with her, she'll be driven to high fury just by the thought of his crushed leather trousers, say, and the store he sets by them. Leo can never forget himself for one second. When you meet him, even when you kiss, it's as if there are two of him, one watching. He is staying with Melita – he's between flats at the moment but he'll be going to New York in two weeks, staying there for at least three months. It's not worth him sorting a place out before he gets back, as he says. So here he is at Melita's. Part of her wishes he'd just move in with her completely. He might as well. Instead of him buying a separate flat they could get a holiday home.

Whenever Leo has gone off on a long trip Melita notices this need in her to make changes to the flat, the layout and the décor. She's not sure why, but it's because she's feeling unsettled, she tells herself. This time it's even more drastic, she starts changing things around before he's even left. A week to go and she's already down at the local charity shops with bags of stuff she feels she just can't bear to live with any more. The flat is looking less cluttered after a few of these trips. Melita says she feels she can breathe better, relax more. Leo is surprised but non committal. He's particularly surprised to see Melita's favourite beaded cushions swooped upon and packed off to the charity shop, though as he says, it's her choice. But he hopes she won't be too long in selecting the right replacements, the chairs would be just a bit too uncomfortable without any cushions at all. She says she needs to find cushions that are exactly right. And then she throws out the beige and black rug that kind of went with the discarded cushions and a short wickerwork bookcase from by the door that she had never liked very much anyway. Melita flings out her arms expansively, as though to show how much room there is in the flat now. She says that before she'd thrown all those things out she'd felt constricted here, hemmed in. Leo says he didn't know she'd felt that way, but he doesn't pay that much attention, his mind is already on New York and what he's going on to. That's his usual way. Melita will sort it out while he's away, he hardly gives the matter another thought. He straightens his red and purple tie. It's a tie and suit day. Silk, of course.

Seeing Leo off at Heathrow Melita feels desolate, has the same feeling she always has – what if she never sees him again? Stupid, she knows, but what if? She supposes she must be insecure, goes home instead of out on the town, and starts dismantling her bedroom furniture. It has a crowded out feel, the bedroom, she wants it streamline. The dresser and wardrobe can go. Clothes? Well, she's got far too many anyway, clothes she never uses, that she hasn't worn for ages, that are just slightly out of date. Many of which probably don't fit. Melita throws things out. Stuff she doesn't need but also certain things she thought she'd liked. Now she wants them all gone. Afterwards her space is open and clear, she feels happier although a little lost in it. She walks barefoot throughout the bereft rooms, occasionally wondering what Leo will make of the change. What's nice is there will be just the two of them here, nothing to hide behind, nothing to obscure. In a way it's an entirely intimate idea which lies behind this shedding. Only the two of them left – her and Leo, with nothing to hamper them. They will be together in a space of intimate possibility. They will be so deliciously alone.

The interior of the *TimeShare* chalet is like a doll's house, all the colours are in pastel shades. It's a doll's house for two with everything in pairs. In the bathroom two pastel blue hand towels lie over the towel rail on top of two, bigger yellow bath sheets, the seams all running the same way. In the open plan living area the table is laid with two identical, facing place-settings. *Everything* is in pale blue and yellow. And from the padded placemats to the folded table napkins to the cushions and curtains, everything has a pattern of kites with flying streamers twirling, finishing in a bow. The placemats are blue with yellow kites, the curtains are yellow with blue kites.

At the time they make Melita feel slightly dizzy. The table napkins are crisp and folded into perfect fat rolls which lie next to the yellow sideplates. It's impossible to imagine people here, they would not be perfect enough to fit in with the environment. They would be too fat or sweaty, even the politest would seem uncouth, the neatest would look ungainly. The place is just like a museum where the artefacts were never in use, show pieces not meant for touching; a museum intended to give people a sense of being cleaner and less crumpled than it is really possible to be. So that if they actually were to move in here they would start to feel intimidated and inadequate by comparison. It wouldn't work except as a fantasy, a place to be passed through in the realm of dream. As Melita walked round the chalet, viewing it, a shudder moved through her thinking of how the place would have become in a too short space of time. All the gleaming plastic gadgets set out now in attractive little displays would have turned smeared and tatty, the pale blue and yellow fabric would wear badly and lose its crisp look, the padding would quickly start showing through the veneer of thin shiny cloth. The chalet was done out for immediate effect, that was all, to bring out noises of admiration from strangers as they passed through its rooms. You could see the chemical blue pool from a lacy curtained window to remind you where you were. It was all a dream which could never be sustained, not even in the moment of first experience because it was too twee and already too dated to really be what it was telling you it was.

Melita is meeting Leo at the airport. Nearly three months have gone by since he'd left. He is talkative and pleased to see her, he is loving and relieved to be back. All the way over to Melita's in the taxi, between kisses, Leo is telling her how fabulous New York is, how cool, but with such a fantastically new and now feel to it that it's hard to keep up with. Of course he was made for it, he had no problems, he was the coolest and newest, after all. But still. He is glad to be back. Being with Melita, he says, feels like coming home. He can't wait to get settled in the flat and unwind. New York has a fast pace. He loves that, of course, and it'll be good to go back there, which he *will* do in six months' time. He's been invited and, he freely admits, he has already committed himself. But in the meantime, in the meantime, it will be great just to chill, to relax in a homey place. It's just not realistic to expect to be cool and fast all of the time. He brushes a few specks from his tan suede jacket sleeve, squeezes Melita's arm as the taxi pulls up outside her address. He *is* glad to be back.

John Halladay

Hartwig, Hermann and Hartmut

Hartwig, Hermann and Hartmut are unconvincing,
their façade of decadence is unattractive.
They tie ribbons or daisies around their helmets.
To be different, I mean to get away with it,
one must do more than poke one's paunch at the ceiling
and groan that schnapps is worse than weissbier for the gout
(that is Hartwig). He doesn't have the grace or wit.
Hartmut eats his snot in public. He's disgusting
but he thinks he's cute – as do Hartwig and Hermann,
whereas the rest of us are just nauseated.
Hermann plays his teeth as if they were organ keys
and leaves his trousers open deliberately.
So what, they ask? Haven't they prospered at a time
when everyone else is dead or broken or burned?
Their survival is a grace, it contains its own
beneficence, it parents its own atonement.
They smile at me, brown-toothed, smelly, fat, tight-tunic'd.
They're elegant, they believe it. (Who'd disagree?
They'd be shot, downwind, in a cold railway siding.
The Reich has quotas, so its bonuses are paid.)
Yes they're clever, decadent, and . . . hear how they fart.

The Second Day That Jude Calls It The First Day

The second day Jude calls it the first day
I'm suspicious of his motivation.

"Jesse," he says, "I feel like I'm a conduit between two bottles."
He empties one to make him sleep
then he wakes and has to empty the other.
That there's $90 brandy he's filterin' through his old kidneys.
That and a great white fizzin' wine that
one of Jonah's boys got back from Dallas.
"Think I'll try and kill myself again."
Smoking stogies, no Havanas today,
Jude wants to die an American.

He says, "guessed life was like Wall Street –
a smash then everything'd come right again.
Thought if I could get me a purpose,

I could stop wishing on cancer.
Maybe quit smokin'."

Next day I go look for the body
and the body's still drunk and in no mood to quit it.
With all that licquor and dope
he forgot to load his rifle
before he put it on his teeth.
He was reminiscin' then got so drunk
he misplaced the cartridge.
He don't stop laughin'.
"You was in my condition," he grins through the booze,
"you'd keep practisin' til you got it right,
sure was havin' me a time
rememberin' them times when you and me . . ."

Other times too, I recall,
some of 'em was even good.

Says, he might try again tonite
if'n the mood comes and he can be bothered.

Mementoes of a Great Adventurer

Chap said, "you was decent you'd get a car
same as everybody else that's decent."
I didn't know what to say,
nor, if I'd a put down, how I'd say it.
Me, sorry the train was late and I'd lost my usual seat,
the muffed connection, two thugs at the station a nuisance
then a damp tramp up under-lit roads.
I prefer the country, but even I get annoyed
at the roughness and the noise of it,
the sounds carry (screeches, that sort).
Same chap passed me afterwards -
"buy a friggin' car, cheapskate" -
and he swerved into the ditch.
It was a red Manta, stickers on the boot,
(not of the considerate or ecological kind:
zooparks, consumer deliverables, honk . . .)
He wasn't going fast, slow enough to shout.
I'd say he was dead before I reached him.

John Halladay
A North Cove Evening

Me, I like that story
'bout Goliath and the little shit
who got dumped on.
What's a man?
Small guys with attitudes and big moustaches?
Fat guys, patriots and the friends of patriots?
A good seducer's a man,
a good doctor's a man.
A snotty kid with anti-Corporate cordite on his fingers,
he's a man.
I ain't one for distinctions or discriminations
where they ain't called for.
A man ain't a vision.
A vision's no more'n a way to get rich quick.
A man's less than that.

Heh, what's a man?
I ain't got no determined picture
Only a mixture that I can't connect.

My old daddy done say:
if it tastes like chicken then it's probably human.

Any Pulp's Sufficient, Mulched with Sugar by a Cretin

Minnie compares the pith to the peeling of infinity
and the pips are only angels to be crushed beneath her flails.
Minnie scours the galaxies for fibres of divinity.
She decants the constellations in a hopper full of nails.

Where a deity has moulded its intentions into accidents
Minnie sieves the cosmos through a pair of crusted tights.
Her fingers tease the rind into a compote of indifference
while she pricks out citrus demons for celestial delights.

Minnie steers the future from a maisonette in Gypsyville,
an infinitude of labels on a multiverse of pots.
She's reserved the Maker's conscience in a basin on her windowsill
for a seedless spice confection in which Minnie calls the shots.

The Lord's renounced creation and let Minnie set the map
for God's a rotten draughtsman (and His marmalade is crap).

The Scavenger

The first sign of fear came from the birds. Crows circled, cawing, screaming, spiralling upwards. Starlings followed, shrieking, one dark mass spiralling into the thin grey clouds that had suddenly hidden the spring sun. Aislie stood in the meadow, watching the heaving wings disappear into infinity and wondered what had spooked them. No human being was visible on the farm, the meadows stretching greenly behind her to the farmhouse, a smudged pencil sketch in the distance.

She shivered. The warmth had beckoned her, torn her from her painting, and she had breathed the fresh sweet smell of hedgerows budding, primroses and dewy grass. Father was ploughing the first turn of the year and mother busied herself baking, a domestic scene that had framed her childhood, fettered her now as she longed to escape the solitude of the soft hills, a longing poured into her paintings, paintings of tall buildings, moonswept roofs, neon lights brightly daubed and rows of people, people in the streets at night, people living in the nights, her dreams fed these scenes. She would go there, one day, it was a promise, a promise whispered in dark nights as the wind howled and snow lashed the peaks, a whisper seeping through the cold windows and slipping into obscurity. Each summer when father traipsed the hedgerows, blocking escape routes for the lambs, she saw her dream of freedom bondaged too.

Her thoughts were whirled away with the birds as their cries lessened and fragmented, faint screams silencing and then nothing moved, no bird song piped, and through the grey mist she saw a darker shadow, gliding nearer, grey, yellow-grey, yellow suited and hooded, arms and legs spread-eagled, swaying, swooping to the ground. It was a man, lying inert, flat on his stomach in the meadow.

She stepped nearer as he slowly coiled and sat up. The hood fell from his face and dark curls cascaded to his shoulders. His eyes met hers, green-blue eyes, eyes the colour of the swimming pool, in the shallow end. They showed no surprise at her presence.

"Shouldn't you have a parachute?" She wondered why he wasn't hurt.

He smiled. "Have you never heard of free-falling?"

"What, all the way down?"

"It's not widely advertised, too dangerous, but yes, it's possible."

"So I see."

She felt no fear of the stranger and, as he stood up and freed himself from his suit, she saw he was quite normal in appearance. Older than herself maybe, but sure in his movements, at ease with his circumstances. He folded the suit amazingly small and tucked it into his bag. He stood looking at her, his pale eyes assessing, a faint frown on his brow.

"Well, Aislie," his voice was amused, gentle, "will you come with me?"

He held out his hand and, unthinking, she took it. Walking beside him across the meadow the farm and its fetters fell away and her mind opened to the future.

"You fell badly," Meridon said, watching her as he sat on the bed.

Aislie frowned, her fingers following the line of bandage around her forehead. She remembered the sudden panic, the ground swaying in her vision, her relaxed arms tensing and her fingers reaching forward. Then her swooping descent degenerating into a hellish plummet, the ground relentlessly hard, and she was rolling, hurting and then the searing crunch to her head, shards of lightening in her brain, pain and blessed darkness; until now. She looked around the room. The light was strong, too harsh for her eyes. She winced.

"Where am I?"

"You're at home." Meridon leaned forward and brushed her brow.

Aislie stared at the stranger. "Who are you?"

"Meridon. You don't remember?" She shook her head, fear lurching in her stomach. "We went skydiving, you needed inspiration for your painting. You were lost, ideas had stagnated; we went freefalling."

Aislie leaned back on the pillows, defeated.

"Rest," Meridon ordered. "I'll be back later."

He left the room and Aislie succumbed to the numbness. She was afraid. Dark tendrils of thought drifted into her consciousness. She remembered the birds; great swooping shadows in her mind, wings disturbing, calls shuddering through her being. The birds, she felt the shaking begin again. Meridon must be right, they were skydiving. How else would she have seen the birds?

She couldn't remember. The room was unfamiliar, would she really have chosen such sombre coloured drapes?

And Meridon, did she love him? He had said 'home' and she occupied a double bed; so she lived with him? For some reason the thought terrified her, jarred her reasoning, evoked the same sickening fear that she recalled as she fell, fell through the birds.

'Meridon,' she tried the syllables over her tongue, 'Meridon,' but the name was clumsy to her. What had he said about painting? She needed inspiration? Painting, brushes on canvas, that was a comforting muse, familiar? Maybe. The effort of focusing her senses throbbed through her head and she relinquished her brain to the shadows. She let the dreams overcome reality and slipped into darkness.

"Paintings by Aislie." The banner filled her with pride. Her own exhibition, and in a prominent part of town. Twelve months hard work accumulating in this, and she couldn't have done it without the help of Meridon.

She still wasn't sure exactly how she had met Meridon or from whence she had come to his home. Her memories of her horrendous fall remained confused, but she had ceased to question his answers. All that mattered was her painting. She stood in front of the largest, a spring scene in the country, details taken from vague memories that haunted the grey areas of her mind. She knew it was good. Did it exist, this place immortalised with her brushes? She didn't know and it was no longer important.

"Can't you remember?" Meridon persisted sometimes. She shook her head.

She had asked herself the same question when her brushes had created her first picture. A farmhouse, surrounded by fields, green blossoming hedges, a figure beneath the roses, faint, shadowy.

"I remember nothing. You explained my past, before the fall; how we met here in the city and went skydiving. You hadn't known me long. You can't answer my pleas for knowledge of my childhood; it must have been here in the city, there is nowhere else, no one has claimed me despite my search. Perhaps I have no family. I have to believe you, I have no other truth."

Meridon appeared satisfied with her replies. She loved her studio, alien though it appeared at first. Her paintings were successful and made them a good income, she was somehow surprised by this. Merison was her agent, he informed her, as well as her lover. She accepted this information and concentrated on her painting.

Colours spewed, animals stirred, wind-lashed trees bowed and the air flowed, incandescent through the shifting hedgerows. Her imagination conjured delicate buds, sprayed shafts of ethereal flowers; her heart was overwhelmed with an abundance of joy and she purged it all onto canvas. Her paintings left her exhausted as if her soul had been wrung through her fingertips and splurged for exploitation.

Her exhibition was a success. She wandered quietly behind the viewers, listening to their comments.

"They're so realistic!" The man was studying the farmyard scene, animals feeding, fields forming a backcloth. "You'd think she'd actually seen a farm. She certainly has imagination."

"The history books are pretty good on description. After all, farming was a way of life decades ago; unimaginable to me, but there you are, it was an interesting era."

"Fascinating!" agreed his companion. "It must have been a strange existence."

"That's what all modern generations think about the past! It's difficult to imagine a world other than the one we live in."

"Yes, but all that empty land, animals roaming around, barbaric!"

Her paintings decorated Meridon's great house, there were none like it; until she found the watercolour in the summerhouse. She had wandered in the sunshine through the walled garden that dimmed the traffic noise and offered peace. Flowers bloomed in spring disarray, carefully nurtured in the malodorous air. In the far corner a summerhouse nestled and she pushed the long grasses aside and crept into the dusty gloom.

A grimy table, a forgotten chair, and the picture. She wiped the debris from the glass and the colours thrust themselves into the light. Carefully she carried the frame outside and studied the scene. A river, silver in the sunshine, grassy banks and birds. It was the birds that caught a fragment in her mind. She hadn't seen birds since her fall and there they were, beautifully caught in wing-fluttering movement. She carried her find to the house. She wasn't sure why she was nervous, but her stomach churned with familiar fear as she studied the birds. The dark shadows that hunched on the edges of her mind spewed wafts of terror that flicked through her blood. She set the canvas on an easel and awaited Meridon's return.

"Who painted this?"

Meridon stared at the picture, his body so still she felt the tautness of his perception touch her exposed doubts. His eyes, when they travelled slowly to her face, pierced her senses with shards of menace. She drew a shuddering breath and looked away.

"Aislie," his voice was soft and she looked again at his face. The smile was warm, his eyes gentle and she wondered if her disturbed senses had been mistaken.

"That was painted by a protégé of mine, a long while ago." He took the painting and balanced it against the wall. "She was successful, for a while, then she lost interest; and so, of course, did I. I cannot be an agent to a failure." His eyes devoured the brush strokes. "Where did you find this?"

"In the summerhouse." Her voice trembled slightly.

"Ah!" He let out a deep breath. "I had forgotten . . ." He seemed lost in thought.

"Where is she now?"

He shrugged and cast the painting aside, casually, as if of no importance. "Not here." He took her arm. "Come, we have your paintings to package, ready for collection. We will have to arrange another exhibition, when you have filled the studio again."

She allowed herself to be led away and when she returned later the painting had gone. She was uneasy but afraid to mention it again, and, for the next few weeks, she concentrated on her new collection.

She wasn't sure when the memories began to dim. Gradually, they faded beyond recognition. She found herself painting buildings, streets, people masses. Meridon was annoyed.

"These won't sell, Aislie. There are hundreds of artists painting the world of cities. Yours are famous for their difference."

She searched her mind for detail but the sombre mantle that eclipsed her vision spread insidiously through her brain. Birds, she could visualise birds, great funereal atrocities sweeping their wings through her consciousness, and she splattered them in horrific lesions across the canvass. She would tear the pitiless offerings to shreds as Meridon watched, his eyes carefully veiled, but his quiescence sending familiar dread to her very soul.

"Remember," he would insinuate softly in her ear as they shared the consuming bed, "remember, Aislie, look back in your dreams."

And she'd drift into slumber, pushing her mind open to positive visions, and pray as she slipped beyond reality, beyond the city streets to the celestial night that had once cosseted a farm in the country. It was useless. She studied previous paintings but her mind remained a blank. She became despondent.

"You need a break," Meridon's voice was gentle. "We'll go sky-diving, free-fall, your mind will refresh in the air. Remember the last time, the inspiration that followed, the exhibition."

Aislie felt terror twist her stomach. "I could be hurt again!"

"Not this time," his voice was gently compelling. "This time you won't look down, this time you'll float your arms, it will be alright, trust me!"

'Trust me!' The words seared Aislie's mind with foreboding. He propelled her forward and, shaking, Aislie followed him into the plane. They wheeled above the clouds. Meridon took her hand and together they plummeted from the plane, arms and legs spread-eagled.

He smiled and let go of her clutching fingers. Very gently he wheeled away from her vision, merging into a thin grey cloud that blocked the sun. She called his name but the wind tore the words to shreds of cloud and her heart was filled with fear. She heard birds call and saw crows and starlings circling her descent, shrieking, screaming. They swooped about her, their wind tunnels rocking her movements and then she hit the ground.

It took a few minutes to regain her breath and then she brushed the hair from her face and sat up. The grass was still damp from the early dew and she brushed droplets from her arms. Her head hurt and she felt the warm stickiness of blood on her temple. She had bounced over a tuft of grass, landed against a stone. She spat on a tissue and stemmed the trickle that slid slimily towards her ear. It was only a scratch but she ached and her head throbbed. The grey clouds parted and the early morning sun blazed gaily over the farm. She turned and limped back to the farmhouse.

"Your breakfast's nearly spoilt!" her mother grumbled and placed the plate of bacon and eggs in front of Aislie.

"I'm famished!" She attacked the plate with gusto, a smile on her face. "It's going to be a beautiful day."

Her father grunted as he came through the door. "Five more lambs," he commented in satisfaction. "Healthy too. Have to watch the crows though, circling the field they are, scavenging for the frail ones!"

Aislie left the kitchen and went into the small dining room she used as a studio. She stared at the painting on her easel. Buildings, streets, masses of people. She shuddered and, reaching for the canvas, tore it into thin shreds. Why on earth had she painted such grimness? Her head still ached from her fall and she stared at the blank canvas, her brush poised. She began to paint, dipping her brush and casting bold swathes of black across the skyline.

'Birds,' she thought, 'great crows and starlings, circling,' her brush followed her memories and swept swiftly, 'birds, and lambs, poor weak lambs, waiting to be scavenged.' It was bold, it was good and she felt triumphant and yet, as she watched the carnage develop, she shuddered and her disturbed mind allowed the shadows to permeate her vision as she splashed a final drop of bright red blood.

She was exhausted, her horror exorcised, and she turned the painting to the wall. She filled her mind with the farm at sunrise, dew glistening on the grass, newborn lambs tottering over the tufts and she started a new canvas, a golden glow suffusing the skyline.

"That's more like it!" she sighed and, weary, she put her brushes to soak and let lethargy propel her from the room.

In the kitchen her mother had just put down the phone. "That was Jane Morgan, she says the Council have put an order on their farm. They've got to sell."

Her father frowned. "Government expansion plans! If they have their way they'll build all over the good land. There's too many people to house, not enough room in the cities anymore. Ridiculous I call it. How can we breed animals for food if they take our land? Folks have got to eat!"

"It's all this new thinking," her mother moaned. "Vegetarian. No need for meat soon, no need for animals. It's a sad state of affairs." She sighed heavily and opened the oven door, putting the beef to roast.

Her father snorted in disgust. "Soon they'll be no farms left. Then what will folks do. The countryside will be history!"

Kathryn Moss
Fall

One day you won't remember, but I will,
how, Adam-like, you named the tiny brown
creature that crept along the window-sill:
"Look! A bird-spider!" Rapt, you were gazing down
at a new sight – each leg a jointed splinter
just like a spider's; fluttering, papery wings
like mottled scraps of dead beech leaves in winter.
With the authority not knowing brings
you showed me the thing you saw; revealed the bleached
six-legged newsprint fragment as a being
blessed with strange gifts. Briefly a veil was breached
and I saw through the clear lens of your seeing.
I told you, "It's a moth," but I regret
what, to join us in words, you must forget.

Evolution

I am a white boulder,
a flint
patinated white outside,
inside steel grey like the frozen ocean.
I am quite still and stiff.
I am dry.
You
cling to me
like lichen,
like little circles,
yolk-gold and verdigris,
that change what they embrace
imperceptibly
with furred, feathery alchemy.
If I lie long enough
on this earth
with you clinging to me,
your embrace encroaching
as you hum into my skull,
I may be worn down
into something living,
like soil.

Slugs

In they come, nightly, somehow
sensing when we have taken
our hot vastness away, leaving
smooth vinyl flooring, a scene

for each fresh quest. Why
do they come? Here are no leaves
thick with satisfying sap
for them to grind and digest,

grind and digest, methodically.
To gain the off-white vinyl plain
they have to writhe and sway
their delicate jelly guts

over bristly matting that must,
anecdote suggests, excruciate.
Each night, careful in socked feet,
I peer and find just one, perhaps two,

slowly swaying their v-sign horns
beneath the cupboard doors,
or making across the flat
expanse of polypropylene

towards the cupboard under the stairs,
where they'll ignore the pears
and apples we stashed and eat
nothing but darkness, till the salt

white death falls on them
and brings a dark that's final.
Why do they come, leaving their
silver wetness in intricate lattices

over mats and carpets? Is it the warm?
Do they smell vegetation? Are they just
explorers, the vanguard for some invasion?
They're so slow; we'll never know.

Kathryn Moss

Sullen psalm

Let us now praise obscure women,
who learned to doubt when they were small
and soon became practised at it,
yet still sent their children to school

well fed and clothed by their efforts.
They lived doubting each day, moulding
sameness into many curious
wonders. They spent long hours mending

washing and smoothing what was worn,
dirty or roughened. Though their strong
big hands shaped worlds they threaded doubt
into their lives from the long skein

given for their use since childhood.
Peeling apples they never thought
Eve's curiosity was like
their own slight, unflamboyant faults.

The Queen of the Summer

The queen of the summer has two dogs,
bitches, both plump, their tan hair
brilliantined over fat bodies,
dainty daisychains of nipples peeping
from under their bellies.

The queen of the summer
has a small, fair head,
cropped close, tansy-gold,
smiling sweetly in the rain,
her hippy weeds billowing out
royally.

The queen of the summer has a consort,
tall, bearded, affable,
greeting the commoners
of her bramble-battlemented nettle kingdom,
on her behalf. The people
pet the dogs, and shyly
look for a kind glance from

the queen. She can cure
with a touch of those eyes.

He lifts her up, scoops her
recumbent into his big arms,
to spare her light tread the drag
of sticky August clay. She need
never strive through mud,
although she's strong enough,
because he has crowned her
queen of the summer.

Sue Wood

Hey-Ho Said Roly

If she married him she knew that he might turn back into a frog, or possibly a toad. The vicar had stressed the uncertainty of cross-species transformations. "Infinitely migrating protons," he had mimed with the hand gesture that Clarinda had seen when he did the Lord walking on water during Sunday Service. He had counselled her to search out Roly's inner self and love this, "For the soul is changeless, my dear." But Clarinda could not take her eyes off her smart, new acquisition: everything just jelly-mould slick, tipped out onto her pillow after just one kiss on the green nose. The after-taste of gravalax without the dill sauce was fleeting, and Roly had heaved into being, his muscles gleaming, his black hair tousled, his pink member erect and circling with perfect homing instinct towards her thigh. Yes, yes, he was perfect. But she would save him up for marriage, so she handed him a unisex kimono which he crawled into like a clump of flag irises and sat blinking up at her with adoring, gold-flecked eyes.

Other girls had been less fortunate with their transformations. Her cousin Alma had lost an earlobe getting in close to a ferret that showed affection but, sadly, only for a supply of Hot Chick Wings. It was always risky, especially as eighty per cent of creatures were quite happy living in holes or nests and never aspired to monogamy and shrink-wrapped meat. And, of course, you could never tell who or what would 'come across,' so Clarinda had opened up to experiment. She found whole-species men boring, either surging testosterone or limp companions. She once eyed up a great Percheron stallion, but he had bitten her very hard on her right nipple when feeling through her anorak for a peppermint and she had thought all the swinging tackle would be a touch over-stated, even if transformation scaled it down. So she had started taking her lunch to Hinksey Round, the old dew pond at the back of Totteridge Lane.

She had not expected to find love, sex or fleeting romance there. It was so ordinary; the water was muddy and polystyrene chip containers floated on the surface. There were mothers with toddlers feeding the ducks and strawberry-flavoured condoms in the undergrowth. Clarinda was taking time out to consider herself. She threw a Wacky Whopper wrapper vaguely in the direction of the litter bin, a breeze picked it up and splashed it down in the pond. Grabbing her umbrella handle, she tried to guide the wrapper to the edge and dutifully sang the old Wombles' song under her breath as an inducement. Suddenly the wrapper stopped spinning and started moving towards her, underneath a neat pair of thighs pumped rhythmically. The wrapper wavered at the pond's edge and then exploded out of the water into her lap. A second pulse and the frog had cleared the nettles and was gazing up at Clarinda through unblinking golden eyes. This was adoration. She knew it from the Wisemen and the Shepherds. A bigger, better thing than sex, she thought. Curving her neck attractively, Clarinda allowed the frog to hop onto her hand. She gazed down at the small creature and felt powerful. She could crush it with her thumb.

The frog blinked at last and with a voice as frail as the touch of wind on the rushes spoke to her, "Take me home, take me home with you! You are neat, you are clean, you are tidy! You lay one little egg each month tucked up where I can't see it at all. I grind all day, all night at the hundreds of eggs they dump like school tapioca all over the pond. The kids are delinquents from hatching. Never listen (haven't got ears). Eat each other, get eaten. I want a nicer life!" So Clarinda gathered him up and let him rest on the delicious curve of her little breasts. He felt like wet blotting paper stuffed up her bra, but she refused to notice that. The sensation of both being adored and rescuing the adorer made her feel giddy, almost orgasmic.

Roly had, of course, needed a great deal of instruction from Clarinda, the Reverend Peeks and Mrs Chumley the home help, before being able to take advantage of his new human form. He preferred to be completely naked which was alright around the house, although a little troublesome for Clarinda's vow of pre-nuptial chastity. The frog genes gave him such good pecs and glutes. But Mrs Chumley would not have it, "Miss Clarinda, it's indecent. He sits on the pouffe just like a lily pad, his legs up under him and it all dangling down in front. I put a duster over it but his lifting gear got going quick as lightning and had the duster stuck up like it was on a broom handle. I don't envy what's coming to you, must have a sperm count of millions!" Clarinda smiled, dreamily, hopefully.

So together they cajoled Roly into pale green Marks and Spencer boxer shorts. He annoyed Clarinda by checking under the chinos and underwear at odd moments as if the clothes could erase his pride and joy. On one occasion, a woman in the Building Society queue had slapped him so hard that the security man tried to arrest him, but Clarinda explained, "He's a new transformation. Just finding his feet."

"Well, love, if that's where he keeps his feet, you'll need a map on your wedding night!"

Roly had shaken out his long black curls and turning to the riveted queue had begun puffing up his chest, stretching his back and opening his wide wet lips. He looked like one of the three T.V. Tenors facing his audience, filling his lungs and savouring his own manliness. Clarinda felt the hot pride of ownership – this was her man! But the moment was brief. A loud penetrating farting noise came from Roly's mouth. His chest expanded, his throat pulsed, his golden eyes dilated and he performed, right there in front of Mr Liddell's mortgage desk. Clarinda felt as if she was the victim of a car crash as the grinning security man led Roly to the door and she walked through the silent, staring crowds.

The Reverend Peeks advised tolerance, "Do not suppress his genetic imprint, my dear. Utilise, utilise, the Lord's creation! Show him how to be a man, but leave the choice with him. He will recognise the higher good and what is base and unlovely in the mere animal will be suppressed. He aspired out of the pond and so is capable of idealism. If he falls short, forgive him, for which one of us has not descended to the animal?" Clarinda went home determined to forgive, that was easy. She had given him some Clint Eastwood movies to watch. Perhaps they would help.

She found Roly, fully dressed, in fact over-dressed as he was wearing her yellow yachting oilskins over everything else, crouched on the window seat watching very intently. The flies were buzzing up and down the glass. Roly's head followed their movements. His hand moved to swat one of them, but, in a tangle of movements, his tongue shot out and reached the fly before his hand. With a puzzled sigh, he let his hand fall and, realising Clarinda had come into the room, wiped the spit marks off the glass with his gloved hand, green golfing gloves.

"What on earth are you doing?"
"Just looking."
"Looking at what?"
"The road outa town."

Roly strained his neck and shoulders into watchful relaxation and, seeing Mr Upton pass the front gate, swung his hand down to his hip, up again, and narrowed his eyes menacingly at Mr Upton's panting dachshund. Pleased with himself, Roly looked winsomely at Clarinda who crunched the video tape underfoot in her hurry to get to the window. A bluebottle wing glittered on Roly's upper lip.

"Why are you wearing all those clothes?" She could see he was sweating.

"My skin is too thin. It needs to hide."

"But you don't like clothes. You told Mrs Chumley to save the rhubarb leaves yesterday so you could lie under them with nothing on. She said you were up to your old tricks again. And you put the washed lettuce out of the fridge down your boxer shorts. In front of her! You know she hates all that."

Roly turned to face her. "The birds are building nests and the grass is singing as it grows again. It is Spring and I wait and wait for your egg to fall so that I can hold it close to my belly and watch it grow. But you say we must wait. I can feel the hot winds of summer already. They are here in your house, breathing and scorching through the hot air holes. I was sleek and moist and new-skinned when I came to you. Now I am drying up."

Slowly he unbuttoned the oilskin, took off his shirt, trousers and underpants and stood naked in front of Clarinda. Flakes of skin circled lazily and landed on his socks. She saw the red, weeping patches on his waist where the material had chafed. The muscles sagged, his stomach protruded and his tiny cock snuggled like a snail in the folds of his crotch. Clarinda burst into tears and rushed to phone the Reverend Peeks.

No, the Reverend did not know of a way back from transformation status. Hadn't he advised tolerance and a pure love of Roly's soul? Well, yes, the Church would not look down on a brother and sister arrangement, but wasn't she breaking trust with the poor creature? Clarinda was prepared to suffer for her mistake, but not enough to get into bed with him. She knew all along that transformations carried risks. They had been known to slip back and, at worst, you ended up with another pet, or put it in the zoo if it was fierce or messy.

Clarinda realised that Roly would never manage his transformation properly: he could not grasp the point of human life. To him it was hot, dry, quiet and celibate. But she came to this conclusion slowly, the memory of the newly-hatched man on her pillow took years to fade away. So she vowed to make him comfortable at least.

He took up residence in the bathroom. Mrs Chumley disapproved especially when she discovered his reasons for staying there. "Miss Clarinda, he's sleeping stark naked in the shower cubicle and there's watercress from Sainsbury's in the bath tub. He's been getting tadpoles from Hinksey Round and keeping them in there. Won't let the Ajax anywhere near. And you should look down the toilet! It's full of snails and they get out and up the cistern and into your parlour palm. You should be ashamed Miss Clarinda, letting him slack away when we had him dressed and proper handsome."

Clarinda only smiled. Somehow the small potterings of Roly in the bathroom soothed her. She did more gardening and left the dirt under her nails because the tadpoles were growing up in the basin. She and Roly took them back to Hinksey Round when they had got legs. He tenderly put each tiny frog onto a grass stalk and, murmuring its name, made it jump into the water.

"Bye, Sun-freckle, bye, Weed-dredger, and you, High Leaper, stay put in the nice wet reeds. This is the best world!" And he dunked his elegant white hands up to the wrists in black sticky mud.

Chris Kinsey

An Introduction to County Mayo

1. Cottongrass, 1967

Dad parked in a cloud.

I skipped a fence
braved the black bog
for three plumes
of waving cottongrass,
brushed the tufts up and down
my cheek, palm, arm.

"Don't bring it near me child!"
Mrs Burke's smile vanished.
Fading like a headland in rain
she muttered,
"Poor, poor starvation grass…"

Her white head usually bobbed
telling me of homemade
soda bread, buttermilk, barmbrack,
hiding in the fuchsia hedge,
running wild down the mountain.

She wouldn't eat.

In her misty silence
famine came to our car picnic,
her anguish more barbed
than the fence wire which caught me.

I sat very still so no one would see
my jumper unravelling.

2. Camping on Achill Island, 1980

County Mayo trips the whole Atlantic over its doorstep.

Air-hungry soils mop up cloud harvests
with acres of cottongrass.

Tourists, pilgrims and a few retired from exile,
keep shops and bars open.

Most sail away from this diluted land

except the fishermen
in their peat-black currachs
spilling starfish in the harbour.

Wind Chill Factor

A couple coming out of Kwiksave
take their carriers to a flatbed Ford.

The fat woman's wearing a summer dress.
It's October and the shadows stretch
to look up it.

Her hem's set like the floor of a carousel.
Everything hangs awkwardly.
Gravity's not her friend.

They stow groceries on the seat.
A terrier leaps off the dashboard
loops the loop, muffing her arms.

The man brings a crate
plays handrest steadying her climb,
the dog jumps onto the shopping.

She sits, legs splayed on the loadbed,
arms outstretched whilst he lashes her
tenderly to the cab.

When the engine starts
I look at the darkening clouds ahead,
wonder how far they're going.

She's already swede-cold.
I call, "At least give her a blanket."
into exhaust fumes.

Chris Kinsey

Breach of the Peace

A hailstorm sweeps the street again.

Under a rainbow, outside Spar,
a gang of girls duel in text-messages,
toss their heads, cascade hair
and gush laughter.

The lone cop cruises,
a white flag of chip papers
covers his grill.

He slides his window down,
*"Keep the noise down girls.
It's Sunday after all!"*

Silence
except for the kiss of rubber sealing glass.

The girls wait.

The drive-on player exits.

"Fuck Sunday!" ricochets
off every shop in town.

Seeing Yellow
(19th March, 2003)

Early dandelions
splash the verges.

At the edge of the village
men in hard hats
bow to celandines.

An old man with a fist
full of daffodils
halts their digger.

Iraq's sands dust
advancing tanks.

Chris Kinsey

The Night Before Full Moon

The moon is up early
blinking through lashes of fir

it spotlights our walk
then jumps onto the branches of a sycamore

climbing clear of the horizon
it snoops on the sun and blushes.

All we see are planes over charcoal hills
pulling last threads of sunset
through the blueing west.

Leonie Smith

"Congratulations on Purchasing Your Brand New Man . . ."

Inspired by a conversation with Dave "Lovebug" Lee

Sadie had never noticed before; but as she pressed the disconnect button on the phone, she realised how phallic telephones could be. Especially flesh tone cordless ones, such as the one that lay in her hand at the very moment. If this one had a vibrate mode, it could have even passed for a vibrator. She dropped the receiver back in its cradle, and glanced languidly around the sterile environment showroom, with a touch of disdain not unlike a dab of Chanel Number 5 on the wrist. God she hated working for her living. As she smoothed down her off-white suit jacket across her hips, she reflected on how life would be if she were a kept woman, living in a penthouse apartment in the City. Expensive lunches and fashionable clothes, exclusive parties and flamboyant cars.

"Sadie darling . . ." She glanced up from her reverie as Elise the showroom manager strode over from the office doorway, her feet enclosed in a pair of strappy black patent Manolo Blahniks. Such a pointless show of personal wealth, to wear such expensive label shoes to work. "I know it's an awful bore, but I don't think you've noticed that we have a client waiting over by the flat top coupé."

Sadie glanced across and sure enough, between the aforementioned model and the tall lean palm tree just inside the automatic doors, dithered a long-haired dowdy little figure shrouded in a long beige raincoat that as good as brushed the floor. Eyes darting left and right and everywhere, giving everything a once over enthusiastic visual fondling. Sadie sighed heavily.

"Must I?"

Elise nodded. "I'm afraid so, darling. She shouldn't take long. Looks like a straight trade in for one of our secondhand models."

"OK. Warm up the coffee pot, I'll be back in five minutes."

As Sadie approached the client, she fleetingly pondered whether the commission from this sale would enable her to buy herself a diamond watch. The woman flinched as Sadie met her eyes, and she jolted at every click of stiletto heel on the hard white floor.

"Can I help you, madam?" She drawled, unable to suppress a supercilious curl of her narrow scarlet-daubed lip.

The woman's eyes dropped to the floor. "I'd like to make a trade-in," she said, hoarsely, staring at Sadie's feet.

"Madam cannot make a trade-in, unless she has brought an old model to make the trade with." The head raised, the eyes lifted and a flash of quite alluring green dazzled Sadie momentarily, before the head dropped again.

"He's outside." The woman tapped smartly on the window with a bare knuckle and said "Come in, Harry!"

As the model stood fidgetting with his fingers in the middle of the floor, Sadie walked around him and studied him from all angles.

"1947 model, you say?"

"Yes." The woman affirmed. "Been stuck with the miserable git since 1972, unfortunately. He's good-for-nothing. Just comes home from work and slumps into his armchair, waiting for me to bring him his tea and 20 Bensons."

"Dagenham built?"

The model let out a fit of deep chesty smoker's coughing. "Yes."

"His roof needs rethatching." Sadie said, running a careful hand across the model's head. "He's thinned out rather a lot."

"Yes, that's been apparent since I got landed with him."

"How much can he hold?"

"About 40 kilos, but that's become a strain for him since his back started giving him trouble a couple of years ago."

Sadie bent down and looked directly into the model's groin area. "Any problems here?"

The woman blushed but a grin slipped out of her mouth and onto her lips. "He's been misfiring for several years. The rocket doesn't reach the Moon anymore. The tide goes out before the ship comes in. He's not pocketed the pink since, ooh probably when Charlie married Di."

"Any noticable reason why?"

The woman shrugged. "Too fat, too sluggish, too inadequate and just too old. I want a newer model."

Sadie straightened up to her full 5ft 10in and looked directly into the woman's eyes. "Well madam, I'm afraid you won't get much for a model this old and devalued. Women simply don't look for models like this any more. He's out of the Stone Age in comparison to what's available to the single woman in this day and age. May I show you to our 'Used Models' section?"

The woman began to unbutton her raincoat. "That won't be necessary, love." She drew the fabric aside and revealed a slim, lithe figure clung hard by a silver PVC catsuit. "I won the lottery and can afford to upgrade to a better model!" she cried, as she threw the raincoat onto the floor.

"Why didn't you say!" Sadie exclaimed. "Elise! Elise! Bring Mrs . . ." She turned and looked at the woman. "Mrs . . . ?"

"That's Ms. Patricia Lye now. No more Mrs Pat Trubshaw!"

"Bring Ms. Lye a coffee!"

"White, two sugars please!"

Patricia admired the softtop sports model for quite some time, as Sadie stood back and smiled at the probable growth of her commission, far in excess of her expectation this month. She watched Patricia run her fingers lightly across the model's washboard stomach, stand on tiptoes to run her fingers through his soft mousy mass of hair and get a good cupped hand around his 'lunchbox.'

"How old did you say this model was?"

Sadie walked over to the sales desk and leafed through the showroom stocklist. "A 1982 model. Answers to the name of Darren. Is able to iron his own shirts, cooks exquisite Thai food and plays leftback for Chelsea. Capable of slipping you a length of nine inches and has a very flexible tongue."

"I must say, I am rather taken with him. I think I could find room for him in my life without too much difficulty." She sighed. "There's one thing though."

"Which is?"

"He's a bit too new for me. I'd like something a little older, a little more a man-of-the-world."

Patricia's eyes ran lightly across the room, touching upon each of the models where they stood in their various poses across the spartan room, their eyes large with eagerness and one or two of them having more than just a dictionary in their pockets. The harsh studio-esque lighting would have shown up any physical faults upon these taut bodies, but there were none to be seen, no beer bellies, no thinning pates, no hooked noses and, best of all, every last model that stood on that showroom floor packed a full and satisfying lunch *wink wink*.

"What about that one there?"

"The fastback coupé? Let me check his details." Sadie said, as Patricia crossed the floor to stand in front of an exceptionally tall, muscular figure with large soulful eyes and long curly chestnut hair. "He's a 1974 model. Answers to the name of Paul. He's artistic, sensitive, keen on making bold, romantic gestures at short notice; writes and paints in a delicate and soulful manner. Cooks like an angel and has a diploma in plumbing. Oh and he's an animal between the sheets."

"His length?"

"Eight inches."

Patricia clapped a hand upon the model's bum and he turned his head and grinned cheekily at her, displaying a dazzling set of even white teeth. "I like you. In fact I like you a lot. What are his prospects? What is his job?"

Sadie ran her finger down the page. "He's a successful freelance graphic designer with his own company."

There was no hesitation in Patricia now. "I'll take him."

"An excellent choice madam!"

Patricia grinned the grin of the supremely delighted.

"Yes, I think so too."

"He will give you hours of satisfaction, until you decide to trade him in for a newer model."

"Actually, I think I might keep this one for life." She winked at the model, who chuckled heartily.

"If you would care to join me at the sales desk, we will finalise the deal. As I intimated earlier, I'm afraid I cannot give you much for the model you're turning in."

They both looked across at Harry, who let out a ripping fart at that moment. Sadie winced and caught Patricia's eye. "I don't care. I just want to be rid of him."

"I understand."

"What will you do with him?"

Sadie sat down at the desk and gestured her client to the soft leather cream easychair opposite her. "Oh, we'll send him out to the workshop. Our technicians will overhaul and retune him, remove some of his outdated ideas and instill new ones into him. Get him shooting live ammunition again. Hopefully make him saleable."

Another raucous fart made them jump and they both shuddered. "Best of luck with that." Patricia murmured.

"Thank you madam, I think we are gonna need it."

Elise came out of the office, as a beaming Patricia led Paul out of the showroom. Sadie glanced up at her and let out a huge sigh.

"Darling, that was an unexpected sale!"

"Have you seen what she's turned in?" Sadie leaned back almost horizontal in her twirly chair and threw her head back behind her shoulders to stretch. She lifted her arm and pointed in the direction of Harry. She looked up as Elise caught sight of Harry and couldn't help but smirk at the abject horror that filled the delicate face.

"Oh my God. I didn't realise that model was still around!"

"Neither did I."

"Looks like we've got our work cut out for us, then."

"It certainly does." And at that moment, the phone rang. Sadie reached for it. "No rest for the wicked."

"If you'll excuse me darling, I'm going to take Darren out to the workshop and retune him."

"He doesn't need retuning!" Sadie cried, surprised.

Elise arched an eyebrow and beckoned the young model over. Darren smiled as he stepped down from his plinth and Elise held out her hand to him. "Alright, test drive him."

"One of these days, Elise, you're gonna get caught!"

"Maybe, but until then, I'll get my kicks playing with the stock!"

Sadie rolled her eyes as she lifted the phone receiver to her ear. "Studmuffin Man Sales, how can I help you?"

Sean Burn

dante in the laundrette

*its the third circle   where it rains
forever malign   cold & heavy
it never eases   it never changes*
like every place i've been moved on from
& i'm readin dante in the laundrette
fine on this overdue translation racks up
drums ov washing speed or slow
as hub ov heat battles squalls ov hail
which part & sting & slant silver birch
& gulls are so many carrier bags
spewed feral on wind & hurled thru ma
kingdom all towerblocks & tenements

churchless towers huddle in conspiracy
outsized car stereos for the takin   tuned
permanently to uneasy listenin   by now
i'm readin *our minds will go completely null*
as badly worn smalls mediums larges spin
the polycotton mix no longer washin
just like his vowels @ the jobless centre
yoof asks for a light says obsessively
i've seen yer i've seen yer I've seen yer
as security guards enter to empty machines
realise i'm no threat & bid *how yu doin*
pull up ma sleeves & bare slashed wrists

*i've no seen terrorist acts bad as they
penny for halloween eh*   this dull thud
ov fireworks should be 3 weeks away
but the flash ov blue & thump ov powder
is undeniable   *why must yu kick
against the pricks*   why even ask
where memory is lost & dreams the 1st
things stolen i seek redemption thru words
yu ask for miracles   theyre deliverin
oxygen to the 16th floor as i turn
water into urine   go back to yr washin
cleanse stain on yr sheets   cycles done

Sean Burn

mayday

milk crate
takin weight
he hunkers down
to harmonica
bendinscrapin
stretchin realities
in & outta
footsteptime

his 13 stitches
& a scab
where *love*
wz tattooed
mesmerise
this kid in
leathers into
fallin off heels
just when
kevlar cops
come move
'em on

history lessens

in uniform nike
dark as tyne
schools out
& hoardin their
sweets dreams
like theres no
tomorras
in cartoon town
laff as dodgy fotos
ov ashley
are passed round
& fagpacks
in mayfair blue
tumbleweed
thru wallsend
& metros
pass in midair
lordin it over

thicksteak
fishcakes
charity shops
& futures
in the balance
ov 12 year olds
hangin offov metros
shoutin *iloveyu*
without knowin
its coin

      survivors
trainsurfin curve
ov possibilities
1 stop down the line

trans pennine

          in an age ov double-glazin
defenestration becomes twice as hard
& yu ma love had twice as far to fall
than most as i recall while speedin
the a66 which is no route 66 but a more
concrete affair   fast-trackin east
blurrin fields ov rape which werent
there then tho their yellow subtext wz

way back when i fell for yu yr
hi heel beat & in that stiletto moment
ov waitin on yu choosin *sci fi silver*
saw how well yu hid yr difference
& just how subtle yr makeup wz   no
red crimes pinned to us as i palmed
painted dreams small as detonators
across to yu   security never workin
where it went nor the wolfwhistlin lads

             & after
retirin to that caff off the main drag
where they remembered yr makeup
asked who the lucky man wz & refused
payment for our Chinese tea smoky
as stolen pearl i painted on nails
which yu dug in ma flesh as i pulled

Sean Burn

yu ever tighter onto me   mashin lips
like overripe cherries   brushin cerise
tart from yr mouth   we screwed   yu
whisperin how yu never wd never cd
make it as a bloke

                              then rackin up
more ov their infamous patisserie
stuffed with all manner ov mango
strawberry   peach   before dancin out
& across tombstones where we laid
white crumbs for birds across graffiti

i wiped a deeper red off yr mouth
wishin to pour the breath back in

even now tastin yr sweetness

the snake upon ma lips

24:12

pulsin to the bigg markets disco-beatin
a butcher heaves past with bleach as
wannabes crush scrumpy in the gloom
big issues havin hard time pushin
Christmas specials this month ov blue
green pink yellow red blue lights on the blink
as strangers snog like long lost friends
& puffa-jacketed ambassadors
push the latest slot deals to kids
who stomp their freebie balloons
amid this hungerford on helium
body hits deck pretends he is drunk
& fishin pizza from bins   veins
his solzenitsyn beard with mozzarella

& they're moppin down boomroom steps
sweepin out the tsb & petitionin our sex shop
with closure as *its the first thing tourists see*
& lipstick lasses freeze their tits off queuein
for speedbanks goin down   *fightfightfight
fightfight*   we got a regular xmas party
with booze & bruisers & prayin for strippers

Sean Burn

& days white as the driven cocaine
earl greys monumentally pissed off
lookin down on his gunmetal town   til
this woman scatters hemp from her liberty
carrierbag & rollin stones spill outov doorways
  blinded by rainbows & faces in windows
  dya dream @ night   i doubt it

Karin Bachmann
A New Beginning

What am I doing here? Why have I ever agreed to this adventure? I wish I could die!

It started harmlessly enough. A crowd had gathered in front of our town hall, among them my friend Theres. She saw me coming from the shop and waved excitedly. "You've got to read this!"

She pushed me to the blackboard where all the important news gets published. Had somebody announced his wedding? Who had died?

What the people were discussing so eagerly, however, was a large notice:

<u>Wanted</u>
Which young, hardworking woman would like to join and marry me in America? Fare paid. Sincere intentions guaranteed.
Contact Messrs Huber & Gutknecht, solicitors, Aarau

"What a lark!" Theres nudged me in my side. "As if there weren't enough women in America."

"Perhaps he'd like somebody he can speak Swiss to and talk about home with?" I suggested.

"Hedwig, please! What decent woman would agree to travel to America all by herself, engaged to a man she's never seen before?"

I shrugged. What did she know, married and pregnant with her first child and yet four years younger than me?

I am the second of ten brothers and sisters. Traditionally, my parents' farm will go to the eldest brother. We others have to make our living elsewhere. Work is hard to find. The factories are sometimes looking for people but those are badly paid fourteen-hour jobs that will make you cough your soul out because of the soot and fibre in the air. Nevertheless, some families have no choice but to send their children to the factories. It's their job to creep under the looms and mend the broken strings; an important if dangerous task that can't be accomplished by grownups.

My parents, too, were unable to keep all of us at home. There were too many mouths to feed, so they gave my sister and one brother into care. Josy stays with her godfather and Walter with a schoolmate of Father's. Such children are called 'service children' because they are employees rather than family members, and it can be a hard lot. To outsiders this common custom must seem cruel. It's true that Walter and Josy have to work for their living at a young age but this way they don't have to leave school early, don't go hungry and are treated well.

Not all the service children are so lucky. Many are exploited as cheap workers, even ill-treated. Still, as long as there's so much poverty, it can't be helped.

My father told me I could work on the farm until I got married.

When I read the notice, I was twenty-five with still no suitor in sight. The people in the village already called me the spinster. So my prospects were anything but rosy. That night I tossed and turned and did a lot of soul-searching. In the morning, I scraped my savings together, asked Mother whether I could get the day off and begged a lift from a farmer on his way to the market in Aarau.

Huber & Gutknecht were kindly old gentlemen.

"Mister Wenger emigrated to the United States five years ago," they explained. "He owns a farm in California and wishes to share it with a wife. He found that, to use his words, 'The local women are superficial, and rotten workers.' Well, be that as it may, he wants a Swiss wife."

"I see."

"You will understand that we have to ask you a few questions. We take it you've never been married? You're in good health? There's no special reason for you to leave the country? You've never been in conflict with . . . um . . . the law?"

"For heaven's sake, no!"

"Very well. If you accept, you'll receive the tickets to get to San Francisco, where your future husband will meet you, and some money to sustain you on your journey. Do you speak English?"

"No, I don't."

"It might be helpful to take lessons. But you look like an intelligent woman. You'll manage it. Oh, and here is a picture of Mister Wenger. We don't want to push you but we'll need your definite answer within a week."

I took a long look at my husband to be. He was no prince charming. The Prussian moustache didn't suit him at all. I liked his eyes, though. There was a warm, sympathetic quality to them. He looked about thirty-five but the age difference didn't bother me. The young men I knew were either already engaged or have-nots like me. With his farm Mister Wenger could offer me a future. Mister Huber told me Wenger had grown up in the hamlet next to our village, and I thought I remembered having seen him in church and at festivals.

"I'll let you know," I promised and left.

Mother cried when I broke the news to her. Father, although shocked at first, looked at it from the practical side.

"You could die on the way. America is a dangerous place. Who knows what kind of person that Mister Wenger is? He could be an escaped prisoner or maybe he's left another wife and children behind."

"No, he's never been married. I've asked the priest and the schoolteacher. They both remembered him and knew him as a sincere if taciturn man. His entire family died of smallpox. That's why he left."

"Well, I guess a man who can afford more than two hundred Francs worth of tickets plus money for meals and accommodation, not to mention the passport and the solicitors, isn't badly off." And Father gave me his blessing.

"Write to us, will you," Mother sobbed the day I left, handing me a picnic basket that could have fed an army.

Father drove me to Aarau in our wagon. The priest, the teacher, Theres and her family and my family were seeing me off. When we drove away, I turned, waved and shouted, "So long!" which represented almost my entire English vocabulary.

"You could have done worse," Father whispered into my ear when he hugged me goodbye at the station.

Two days in a storm! How can anybody want to become a sailor? I've never felt so sick before. Maybe doing some English will distract me.

"Where are you from? I am from Switzerland. Does you – no – do you speak German? Speak slow, please."

That sentence sounds strange. But then it's a strange language. Sometimes I think I'll never learn it. The pronunciation is particularly difficult. Three days ago, when I was still able to eat, I wanted to pay the steward a compliment. I said, "Fis foot ist rally dilicous," but he didn't understand me. Perhaps he doesn't speak English either?

"I am, you are, he she it is, we are . . ." At least the conjugations are easier than in Swiss and there seem to be fewer exceptions to the grammar rules. I'm not the first one who's had to learn another language; I'll cope.

As soon as the worst of the storm has blown over, I'll go on deck. I need fresh air. Ida will certainly accompany me. She's from a village near Berne and we met in Amsterdam.

What an intimidating place that was! I didn't know such huge cities existed. The biggest place I had seen before was Aarau, which in comparison appears tiny. For the first time I experienced what homesickness was; all alone in that city, a stranger who didn't speak the language, didn't know the money and even less her way around.

I found out that they had cheated me with the exchange rate for the boarding house bill, but what could I have done? Overall I was lucky. I heard about people who lost all their money to touts. There are crooks who specialise in selling the most ridiculous gadgets to guileless emigrants.

I was so happy when I met Ida and her family. They, too, were glad to find somebody who spoke Swiss and was in the same situation. We became friends at once and vowed to try and keep in touch. I gave Ida my address. She didn't have one yet but promised to send it to me as soon as she knew it.

Ida's family is participating in the government's emigration scheme. Some clever politician found out that it costs less to help a family to emigrate than to provide for them in the poorhouses. They give you the tickets, a small sum to help you over the first few weeks, their blessings and off you go. Most families settle in Brazil and Argentina but some opt for the United States.

Poor Ida. I have a place to go to and a husband waiting for me. Like that it will be easier to grow roots. Ida has a husband, a sick father and two small children. For them it must feel like jumping without knowing where they will land.

They say that in America the gold lies on the streets. I don't believe it. It won't be any different from the way it was in Switzerland. (I especially say Switzerland, not home. California is my home now.) If you want to achieve something, you've got to work for it. I'm willing to work hard for a bright future.

I know I will be happy. My husband and I will love each other and have many children. Our farm will be a success and maybe, one day, I'll be able to send some money to provide for my younger brothers and sisters at home – in Switzerland, I mean.

Gordon Hodgeon

In The Purse

Lost it years ago, I never guessed
it slipped straight down between the lining
and the leather, lay low, flat and stiff
as kids in long grass, playing dead.

Got tired of looking for it, thought it best
obliterated with one wipe. I let
the dust put coats on sills, on lintels, breath
that counted to ten thousand while you hid.

Ready or not. Up cracked stairs. Our almost
empty room. Cupboard jammed with the damp.
Swaddled in mildewed, moth-chewed fur
your mother wanted me to wear, I never did,

the purse I carried at our wedding. Twist
the rusted clasp, could get my fingers burned
but push them down into the frayed silk seams
and find it, sick of being sought, not glad

to have its boniness fished out at last,
a grey-faced relic from its shabby shrine,
lining and leather. Love, was that all –
your name on it – it was, I ever had?

Freeze

Think of yourself as a glacier by all means, the progeny
of deep winter, will give a reassurance in the coldness,
the solidity, the hands-off-me slippiness of surface.
You will not though be able to deny that there is movement

and that it is towards me, inevitable, the ice's
pull downhill, out from the cold core, off to where it finds some
    warmth,
and that this movement at its adventurous extremity
melts to a flow that is simply water and feeds springtime.

Not so simple. If the earth is cracked in the head, infected
or insane, poisoned, made war on, if it's in raging fever,
what can save you from liquidity, from the defencelessness,
the wetness of love? Or rescue me from the weight of such tears?

Trying too hard. Only a lump of flesh that's past its freshest,
that grows chill across the shoulders, at the softness of the back,
as in a damp night late in my years I write and cannot know
what gets by through the thin air to where you may not feel the cold

or where you sit inside the mind of a new house, whether you
are making order of so much snow, packing it into chests,
loading the shelves with it, reading its not to be deciphered sounds
or playing them on refrigerators, the silent white keys.

Circular

That morning was so dark, it made me shift
to raise the blind, it was the sky. So far
so good, and then they dropped with dead flies' drift
through the door's slot, first shots of festive fare
from friends who scratch my grudges every year.

Don't need to open them, watch it go by
the weather out there, listen to the clock
cough, you know their parents died or will die
soon enough, or they've split up, but will attack
once more their wed address list, sound heroic.

My age and literate, what's to be done
but writing out last year's disaster list
and demonstrating how to cope and grin
when genius kids are middle-aging fast,
poor specimens of what the future's passed?

They're managing, not companies or gangs,
but getting by, and they are keeping jolly
as muscle shrinks, as joints give out, most things
work with a something aid, and gradually
plastic and steel replace the flesh's folly.

Their celebration is that they survive
and I'm supposed to raise my glass to that,
treasure their trips in photographic trove,
sundown safari or the cruise round Crete.
You have to see the sunny side of fate,

Gordon Hodgeon

I guess, to be a golfer, bash your balls
across some crimplene cow-cleared meadowland,
or go to adult ed., sit in cold halls,
empty your flask while cluttering your mind
with stuff the temporary staff don't understand.

If, it's not likely, any of them read this
and take offence at my ingratitude,
they may well think that I'm taking the piss,
finding their kind intentions misconstrued.
My lifelong learning is in being rude.

Putting it blunt, a card will do next time,
merry old mash, happy new mish, such shlock,
which is all that I need to hear from them
on the other side. It's a piece of cake,
a candle, somebody there when I knock.

Zero

Look at it like I showed you,
like a photograph, you have to
keep on choosing what to put
in your little dancing handbag
stapled to a snow wall
anything could penetrate anytime just
there. Smart, that third dimension,
splits kisses, rips nails.

You stiffened like ice cream
to my freezer fingers
in your cardboard pyjamas,
there was a hint of melting,
of berry juice slices,
a taste at the far end of the signal's range,
maybe a 747 going down unauthorised,
breath knotted in bellies.

Trees smashing light back,
salt sprinkled on leaves, rubble
of angels, the water building
itself down, a white wax candle
that can fuck granite
and does. Hold me responsible,
that edge of rock, that drop in the eyeball,
scratches in a cold blue.

Gordon Hodgeon

Notice

Off for the winter, are you? Bloody hell!
And with old you-know-who along as well?
No need to add explanatory text,
just leave me wondering what you'll tell me next!

Not that I've ever fancied winter sports,
the snazzy awful clothes, the grim reports
of avalanches, all that après-ski,
this is the stuff brings out the worst in me,

the opposite of all the things you like.
When fear kicks in, the nice parts go on strike,
you told me what they were once, can't recall,
but winter sports craps white-out on them all.

You look as if to say you'd thought I might
go thick-eyed as a damp November night
and typically forget to think that spring
will come and you with it, appearing

like what's-her-name from out the underworld,
your face all sun-tanned and your legs unfurled.
I don't forget. If looks could resurrect,
I'd melt the sodden lot, leave winter wrecked,

have all its sports slopped soggy down the drain,
so I could live full-time with you again
in light and warm and dry, not give a shit
what happened to the global warming bit.

You could snap back there never was a time
when we had that arrangement, but your rhyme
to my disgruntlement's infantile myth
is softer, subtler, telling me the truth

and that it's seasonal, its ebbs and flows,
synapses, snaps, stanzaic body-blows
are hymns to love, antiphonal, at odds
with what we dream of snatching from the gods.

As usual, you'll persuade me that's the way,
I'll start the countdown day by bloody day,
hoping next spring and summer lie ahead,
knowing each one is one less till we're dead.

Ruth Henderson

That to Odin

THE VALKYRIES
Running across the heavy wooden drawbridge made Adam sound like a big lad but he's only eight, small for his age and skinny. He has thick black hair, wide blue eyes and his ears stick out. He'd been playing football but before he had time to throw his backpack through the kitchen door his grandmother called from upstairs.
"Go and get Sam. By the time she gets that horse bedded down it'll be dark."
"Right Gran." Adam ran off to fetch his sister.
His Gran's house is inside the walls of an old castle, on the edge of a high cliff. Inside these walls are the ruins of an ancient priory and tombstones of the Kings of Scotland and England, who'd been buried there hundreds of years ago.
At the cliff edge Adam yelled, " Sam, you've got to come in."
She was too far away to hear him.
He shouted louder. "Sam. Sam."
Sam rode faster and faster, urging the little pony along the beach.
Adam huffed to himself. He'd have to fetch her. In a torrent of pebbles and soil he slid down the steep cliff and at the bottom he lay on his back to catch his breath.
There was something odd about the sea. A strange red mist was rolling in with the big breakers. He could see shapes in the mist, shapes of horses. Pushing himself to his feet he realised they really were horses. Big black horses with red eyes and golden hooves and on their backs were girls with white faces and long red hair streaming out behind them. The girls were dressed in fur with tight leather caps on their heads and they carried golden spears.
The horses thundered down, skimming the waves and swooping across the sand. Faster and faster they galloped. Then, right in front of Adam's eyes, they took Sam away . . . into the blood red sky.
Stumbling and slipping over the sea weed Adam screamed for his sister, who was trying to jump from her pony, but she was too high up. The speed of flight took his breath away and suddenly, in a flash of golden lightning, they were gone and Adam was left alone on the deserted beach.
Adam's not sure he's seen what he thinks he's seen. On his hands and knees he crawls up the cliff and still watching the empty sky he stumbles back through the ruins he's played in since he was a baby.
The ancient Priory is his adventure playground and he knows it well. He's certain that through the broken archway the ground is paved with cracked stones and the broken walls reach into the sky because there's no roof on the Priory. At least that's what he would have told you if you'd asked him one nano second ago. Now, he's standing inside

a church. A proper church with a roof, walls and an altar with candles and a golden cross on it. In front of the altar, brown-robed monks are praying.

He looked back the way he'd come and everything seemed the same, just grass that needed cutting and crumbling walls. "This is bad," he mumbled to himself. "This is seriously weird." But he thought that going into the spooky church was the only way to solve the mystery so he crept behind the wooden pews and slipped quietly through an open door.

A full moon rising over the sea gave Adam a clear light to see by. All around him the Priory was intact in every detail. Some stone buildings were built on the cliffs. Adam looked in a few but they were deserted; jobs, like preparing a meal or mending sandals, waited for the monks to finish prayers and return to their duties and the graveyard was as silent as a grave. The last building was the biggest. Like the others the door was unlocked. Adam stepped inside.

He was in a dark, narrow hall.

He tiptoed forward. In the gloomy passageway closed doors made this a dangerous place to be sneaking about. If someone opened a door he'd be discovered and never work out how to find Sam or get back home.

Suddenly he stiffened.

Stood still as a statue.

A handle on the door to his right was turning.

Rooted to the spot Adam couldn't move to save his life.

The door swung back and in the dim light of a flickering candle a tall, robed figure with a hood over its head reached out a hand and its bony fingers closed like cold iron around Adam's wrist.

ODIN

Samantha was terrified. She shouted. "Let me go." But the women ignored her. She tried to get her little pony to turn back. "Whoa! Whoa Faxi! Stop!" He ignored her too. They galloped for hours and hours until they came to a snow-capped mountain where they dropped out of the sky. The wild girls rode away. Sam urged Skinfaxi back up but he threw her and galloped after the devilish animals. Wincing and rubbing her bottom she looked around. She was in a meadow lush with grass and flowers.

The wind blew down and kissed the flowers. It said, "These are my friends. Treat them kindly."

Sam had never heard the wind speak but it felt like a good thing. "Thank you, I will," she answered. In front of her is a giant tree with stags eating the soft leaves, squirrels running up and down, birds flitting and twitting and on the topmost branch was a huge eagle watching over everything. On the grass, in front of this tree, sat a man.

No ordinary man, this is the biggest giant of a man Sam has ever seen. Like the girl riders he has red hair and, despite the shadow cast by the branches, his eyes glow blue. He wears animal skins and beside him is a long golden spear.

Sam steps forward but just in time she realises that a deep chasm cuts right through the ground. Peering cautiously over the edge she jumps back in horror. A huge serpent with three hissing heads is coiled around the roots of the tree and three of the ugliest old women Sam could ever imagine are boiling something in a big, bronze pan, sending up a stink bad enough to choke a dog.

Sam runs but she stumbles over a rock.

A deep, rumbling voice offers help. "Come child. Give me your hand."

Sam looks up at the giant man from the tree.

"Can you read?" he asks.

Sam nods.

"Come then."

Even though she doesn't move Sam finds herself walking beside the man and they are going back to the tree. "No! Stop it!" She tries in vain to pull away. "This is kidnapping! You'll go to jail for this. My mother will sue you! My Gran will slap you! Leave me alone!"

The man bent his head to look at her. "You're brave. I admire that in a warrior."

"I'm not a warrior." Sam was angry.

"A pity. You'd make a fine warrior." His big voice shook the trees and echoed like thunder among the rocky peaks of the mountain.

"Let me go!" Sam demanded. "I didn't ask to be brought here. I was stolen by a pack of smelly witches."

"They're not witches, they're my Valkyries," the giant said.

"Whatever," replied Sam.

"They ride the battlefields and bring me the souls of brave warriors. When I fight the Last Great Battle I'll need all the brave warriors I can find."

"Who are you!"

"I am Odin."

"Odin?" she said, sarcastically. "Odin! Like in the god Odin?"

"I *am* Odin, father of all the gods."

Sam tried to pull away but a powerful force kept her close to Odin. "Let me go." She swung a punch at him but her fist bounced off an invisible wall. "I'm not supposed to speak to strange men, and they don't come much stranger than you."

She tripped, falling to her knees, then softly, from nowhere yet everywhere, she heard the whisper of voices, the merest suggestion of sound that was so unreal she wondered if she was imagining it. The sound floated into her ears saying, "Do not trust him." She looked around but only the pretty, meadow flowers nodded in the warm breeze.

"Was that you?" she asked the flowers.

"No," they said, tossing their heads.

"It wasn't me either," said the breeze.

Odin yanked her to her feet then strode on, continuing the conversation. "It makes no difference if you believe me or not. What *you* believe can't change anything. On the other hand what *I* believe can change the world." This made him laugh.

Sam wasn't amused. "Fine if you say so. Now, if you're so clever, wave your magic hammer and send me home."

"Spear. I have a magic spear and a belt. Thor has a hammer."

"Whatever." Sam didn't apologise.

Picking Sam up, in one hand, Odin stepped across the chasm sending the serpents hissing and the crones howling. He dropped her on the grass then threw himself beside her.

"Ouch," the grasses all cried.

But Odin was ignorant of their pain. "You told me you can read," he said.

" Of course," Sam told him.

"If you reveal Knowledge to me I'll return you to your time. I always keep my word. I am an honourable god," he boasted.

"He is a liar," the whispering voices told Sam.

She looked around but still there was only the tree, the grass and the flowers.

"Are you sure it's not you?" she asked the grasses again.

They shook their heads, sending pollen tumbling through the air and making Sam sneeze.

"I've gone mad," she told herself. "I must have fallen off Skinfaxi and bumped my head." Discovering that she was no longer bound to Odin's side she paced about trying to find who was doing the whispering but there was no one there.

After a while the long, low note of a horn came from far away, echoing around the hills and up the mountain.

Odin jumped up. "They're here! My warriors are bringing me a magic Book that will show me the future. But it will be in a language new to me. If you tell me what the book says I'll release you. You have my promise." He bent down until his face was close to Sam's. His blue ice eyes were evil and his breath froze in the sunshine. He terrified her. "But if you fail you'll sleep under the mountain with the Valkyries. Forever."

THE MAD MONK

The tall, hooded figure had pulled Adam into the room. He turned him to face the corner. "Stay there awhile and think about your sin," he mumbled in a quiet voice.

"What sin?" Adam knew he hadn't done anything wrong.

" Silence!" commanded the man.

Adam sneaked a look around him. The room had a high ceiling and big window arches with no glass in them. One wall held shelves of books and in the middle, on a long table, candles flickered in the draught. The man, who was only a monk, had his back to Adam and was busy writing. In front of him were bottles of coloured ink. Adam stepped closer. The monk stayed hunched over his work. At one end of the table a package was tied with string and sealed with red wax. Beside it a pile of loose pages lay on a scrap of leather. The colours were so bright that even in the poor light of the moon and candles they shone brilliantly. The letters were etched in gold and filled in with red, blue and green. Patterns wove up and down the edges of the pages and pictures of animals and birds decorated the writing.

Adam had been to Durham Cathedral to see the Lindisfarne Gospels, books written by monks hundreds of years ago. He thought that these must be them. "Wheeow," he whistled.

Without lifting his head the monk spoke. "It must have been a very little sin if you have pondered it so quickly."

Adam jumped back to his corner.

"Come close boy," the monk invited.

Adam walked towards him.

The tall figure turned around and pushed back the hood of his robe. He was thin and pale with dark hair cut in a ring around his almost pointed head and he peered at Adam as if he needed glasses. His long, bony fingers were coloured red and blue from the inks he was working with. "Why were you sent to me? What is this infinitesimal sin?" He measured a narrow space in the air between his red thumb and blue forefinger.

"I haven't done anything. I'm looking for my sister," Adam told him.

The monk grinned showing broken yellow teeth. "Ye'll find no maidens in these walls."

"You don't understand. Some women came down from the sky and took her away and . . ."

The monk interrupted. "The Valkyries?"

"Beats me," said Adam. "What are valerys?"

"Valkyries. They come with the Vikings to carry the dead to their blasphemous palace in Valhalla. Have ye seen their ships?" He leapt up to peer through the tall windows.

"Er no," said Adam. "No I don't think so."

"Dolt!" The monk whacked Adam across his head with his bony hand. "Ye'll be murdered in your bed with such carelessness." His robe billowed around him as he whirled past, running up and down the length of the table, gathering together the loose pages of his manuscript.

"They're the Lindisfarne Gospels aren't they?" Adam asked him.

The monk pointed his hooked nose at Adam. "How do ye come to know about the Gospels?"

(*Ho, thought Adam, you'll never believe it.*) He invented something. "I mean I've heard about them."

The monk nodded. "I too have heard about the work of my brothers on the Holy Island of Lindisfarne but these pages are my own poor effort. These are the Shieldsmouth Gospels."

"From what I've seen these are just as good." Adam complimented the virtuous man.

"Ye have seen the Lindisfarne Gospels!" The monk was worried. "Are ye in the pay of the Vikings?" His words ended in a scream and suddenly this gentle man-of-God grabbed Adam by the neck and shook him. "Creeping about in the dead of night spying. Ye'll be thrown into the sea for such treachery." He dragged Adam out of the Scriptorium and down the passage, then to the cliff edge where the gulls screeched in protest at being disturbed. In a towering fury he snarled, "I will not have my work stolen by a boy."

Adam choked as the monk's fist tightened around his soft, skinny neck, lifting him off the ground. The monk was glaring at him, his mouth drawn back in a snarl, his eyes wide open and rolling around. Adam was scared stiff. He tried to yell out but he could hardly breathe never mind talk. He kicked out with his legs, punched toward the monk with his puny little fists but it did no good. In fact he thought the monk had forgotten Adam was dangling at the end of his arm, he was staring out to sea.

Suddenly he realised what a terrible thing he was doing to a small boy and muttering to himself he pulled Adam onto the grass and straightened his shirt.

Adam managed to speak. "I don't want your books. I just want to find Sam."

The monk was staring down into the little bay where the sea swirled into a moat that encircled the castle. Riding on the waves were two longboats full of fearsome men in furs and steel helmets. It was obvious to Adam they were Vikings.

He'd been to the Yorvik Centre in York and these men with their shields and spears, glinting in the moonlight, were exactly as shown in the museum.

"Sound the alarm. Sound the alarm," The monk shouted, running to where a sleeping man lay curled up under a tombstone. He kicked the man awake. "Light the beacon you useless layabout."

The man jumped up and set alight a prepared bonfire held in an iron brazier.

From every door monks came running, calling instructions, carrying precious treasures and fleeing to the castle gates.

Adam followed the monk back into the Scriptorium where he was bundling his precious pages into a sack then he thrust the package into Adam's backpack and dragging Adam behind him, ran to the castle gate. It was too late. Their escape was cut off by the madly yelling

Ruth Henderson

Vikings who were surging across the drawbridge. They cared for no one. With their heavy swords they slashed at monks, scholars and workers, who all fell dead in their tracks. They set fires and ransacked the church and outbuildings.

The monk turned down a shadowy path under the castle walls. The path got narrower and darker. The monk stooped his bony shoulders and crept under a bush of thorny branches then disappeared from view. Adam followed him. Down and down through the rock. It was pitch black and he kept tripping over the uneven floor and when he put out a hand to steady himself, it came away wet. Shaking with terror Adam realised that he was following this crazy monk into a secret passage that would take him two thousand years away from his own time.

Convinced that the Vikings had more chance of leading him to Sam than the monk, he shouted, "I have to go." Cold dread poured over Adam as he peered into the empty darkness then with a deep, bone-shuddering breath he turned back to the madness of the Viking raid.

Daphne Rance

Mrs Linden

"Mrs Linden died last Sunday."
You know how these things slide about
A village, slip between houses, down alleys!
There's an alley past her garden so I walked that way
Today. I didn't know her, had never even seen her,
Only seen long pink knickers pegged to a piece of string
By her back door and the door swing and a blare of radio tunes
Fall out, fall past her old deaf ears I guess,
Into the dank garden.
March is a poor time to die for any one –
Raw in the chest and your feet cold in bed.

The garden hadn't changed since I last went by.
There stood the clothes line, neatly folded under its green cover.
I'd never seen it used but the grass round it
Was always cut by someone and the same someone, I supposed,
Dug the small patch in the opposite corner every year
Re-fixed the bean-poles and planted out the beans
In two neat rows. They grew well. I used to judge mine
Against hers and hers were best,
But I doubt she ever picked them. The old pods
Still rattle there blackened with rot. The rest is wilderness
But primroses splash across the weeds like dappled sunlight
And I have seen, among her nettles, the finest lilies blaze.
I walked round by her front door, thinking the funeral
Would leave its traces. But no, the drift of dirt still dumbed the step
Blown off the road by old winds,
Swags of smutty cobwebs still sealed the cracks round the red door.
The coffin must have gone by the back way and her dying
Has made no difference at all.
Except perhaps to the someone who dug her garden.

The Woman In A Red Dress

The woman in the photograph looks, as I expected, old.
Not so much the arms – I foresaw
That her flesh would hang limply on the long bones – it is the right hand
Pitched tense against the smoulder of her dress
Bones visible from wrist to claw
And sharp knuckles humping the skin. You saw
How a touch would ruckle it – the blotched, translucent membrane

Daphne Rance

Inlaid with its burden of blue filaments
Carrying, in slow beat, her blood.
I have seen that same eagle's or lion's paw carved proud in walnut
On fine furniture as a man's masterwork.

Her eyes in the photograph look inward, not meeting yours
But turned as by a mirror to look instead
Down into herself. Is it dark there or only
Infinitely deep? It is not a route you may follow.

Her lips are thin, having lost ripeness to Time's kiss. However
She does not need your pity, she is whole
For there is one man who knows the tenderness,
The warmth and laughter in her and the increment of moments.
She rests content.

City Street In Spring

The street is a canvas
And the hand working.
It is sketched in with a cross-nibbed pen
Scratchily, hastily; blots where heavy bodies, slowing
Run together and let memories butt into single globules;
Then speed-lines skitter into interrupted tacks
Taking off across temporarily numbed traffic.

The flow gasps, grabs breath again and surges –
This way, that way.

Half-lost in the wash of a brushful of white noise
New streaks break out
Intensifying from thick pigment to threads
That are flipped and tagged into faces,
Blackened to hair or the snagged edge of a beard
Or a dog-lead or the heavy hang of a bag
From some angular shoulder.

Ink-hard scratch-lines of angry eyes shout what I can't –
Don't want – to catch, and the smudge then of a dozen
Others in charred light fades
Away under patch-stemmed, twiggy-headed planes
With their exact, black cherries swinging
Against etched porticoes and the horizontal shadows of steps.

Even here blown petals
Fall delicately out of the air.

Daphne Rance

Studying The Architecture

Lay a foundation stone
Or a word on paper:
'Archway'
      (Entry
      Shadowed
      Keystone
      Unknown
      Cool)

Or 'Wall'
      (Roughgrained
      Skinwarm
      Harbourage
      Obdurate
      Anchored
      Tough)

Or perhaps 'Roof'
      (Ridged
      Wrinkled
      Mossed
      Straddling
      Bright)

The enclosed space enfolds light
Stores it in warm stone
Nourishes roses and marjoram
Holds silence when the moon
Spills sheet silver
Over
The earth floor.

'Earth'
      Pudding-rich
      Deep underfoot
      It will endure
Paved for the blue velvet slippers of my lady
And her knight's spur.

Daphne Rance

Nowadays

Her chair faces the window. The sparrows
Are her family. She knows the soft ruffling,
The abasement, of the young ones begging titbits
And the cock's enthusiastic demonstration of a hunting father
And refusal to be drawn. The spike of yellow mullein is one source of
   their insects.
She gauges its growth daily against the shed's roof. The shed
That opens away from her, that houses bicycles and prams
And before that the tin bath, perhaps the wash-copper bricked in,
Coal, spuds or even the holed board over stinking buckets.
Her own house has no outplace. It is not busy like that.

She eats soup. She has put the bread on a sideplate only because its
   raised rim
Is good for holding the book open. Meals would be lonely
If she had nothing to read, no to-and-fro of arguments in her head,
No views laid out like lakes and forests below her vantage point
On the mountainside. When she thought about it like that
It meant she was escaping from the endless todays
Hung around her like beads on a necklace.
Sometimes she imagined the colours of beads: moonstone and opal,
All the pearl colours – rose, cream, soft gold, even what they call
   'black' pearls
Or the clear-water the feel-of-swimming aquamarines.
You could twist and slide them along their cotton,
Run them again and again through your fingers,
Round and round, endless like todays and todays and todays.
It's not that her days have no beauty in them
Though it's mostly outside the window, where things grow and
   change –
Seagulls soaring on the lift of the sky, blue butterflies.
She supposed that to be warm enough was also a sort of beauty
And to have food to eat and water in a twisting rush when you turned
   taps
But O how she longed to break this chain of days just now and again.
Nothing ridiculous, just go to the Cream Teas in The Grange garden
On the fifth of August, or be driven somewhere in October
Past banks of flaming beech trees and the sea.

She ticks through the list of friends she knows well enough to dare
To ask to take her. Each year it needs more daring.
And anyway these young people have children and husbands
Who come before her. So busy nowadays.

Josephine Fagan

Venus on a Soap-dish

We were meant to come to Italy ten years ago after we got married but Tom couldn't get time off work. He calls this trip our second honeymoon.

"You go ahead," he barely lifts his head from the pillow. "You know I'm not a great one for art galleries... I'll just have another forty winks... I could meet you at that little café we went to last night... say about twelve..."

I arrive at the Uffizi just as it's opening and sign-up for the full guided-tour. Having ushered us upstairs, our guide assembles the group in front of Botticelli's *Birth Of Venus*. After a short pause, he theatrically clears his throat. Appreciative sighs and mutterings are stifled. Only when he has complete silence does he begin. First he draws our attention to the painting's central figure – a naked woman perched on top of a large scallop-shell. "See? Having risen from the waves, the goddess of love is gently blown ashore by the wind..." He enthuses over her long yellow hair and languid curves then crosses the gallery. "And now we will look at Botticelli's *Primavera*." Pointing to a group of dancing figures, he singles out the same pale woman for scrutiny, "Notice how he uses his muse again and again... now she is one of his *Three Graces*..." Before we proceed to the next room, he pulls a dog-eared postcard from his jacket pocket and hands it round. "This is the great master's *Allegory of Calumny*... Look closely, in this picture he has used her to represent *Truth*..."

When the tour is finished, I walk round the whole gallery again on my own. This time I save Venus till last. Serene and unmoved she smiles into the distance while a never-ending stream of tourists continues to ebb and flow beneath her.

Outside, the midday heat is stifling. Trying to make the short walk to the café last as long as possible, I stroll the narrow cobbled streets of Florence. Lingering over markets stalls and shop windows, I scrutinise souvenirs, shoes, handbags and a whole host of things I know I will not buy. As time passes, I become increasingly unsure of my bearings. I turn into a featureless alleyway – now only half confident of my route to the café. It all looks so different by day. Just as I'm about to retrace my steps, the street fans out into a familiar sunlit piazza. Bleached stonewalls enclose a central fountain which is still sadly dustbowl dry. Last night's courting couples have been replaced by children and mothers who walk by hand in hand. Young men on mopeds buzz past leaving hot blue comets of exhaust fames. On the far side of the square, a group of girls stand talking. Dressed in citrus colours, their bodies seem to sway like exotic blooms in the heat-haze.

The pavement café is almost full. Tom doesn't seem to be there. Finding a vacant seat, I look about me, checking each table to see if I've missed him.

Sophisticated regulars signal orders with a nod, or a gesture. Balancing heavy trays on their fingertips, nimble waiters weave in and out between diners. It doesn't really matter that I can't attract their attention – I'm sure Tom will be ages yet. I try to read but the glare from my guidebook's glossy pages makes it impossible – even with sunglasses. Just for once, I wanted Tom to be waiting for me. Shielding my eyes, I look out across the square to see if he's coming. Instead, I see a woman with hair like Botticelli's Venus – like a golden waterfall tumbling over her shoulders. There's something strangely cool and Nordic about her. As she approaches the café, she seems to glide towards the table – as if she too is being borne up on the crest of a wave and gently washed ashore – all that's missing is the curved scallop-shell underfoot. She takes a seat at the unoccupied table adjacent to my own.

Surreptitiously, I angle my chair towards her – the resemblance is remarkable – perhaps this woman is a descendant of the artist's original model. I've never thought Botticelli's Venus looked especially Italian. I almost said as much to the Uffizi guide but maybe there are lots of blondes in Florence. We only arrived yesterday.

Flicking her hair with the back of her hand, the woman takes a pack of cigarettes from her handbag. She leans back on her chair and crosses her legs. A keen-eyed waiter materialises at her elbow. Head half-bowed he attentively lights her cigarette, puts a fresh ashtray on the table and then takes her order.

"*Espresso*." On her lips, the word sounds like the name of a fast train.

The waiter returns in an instant with a tiny cup of strong black coffee. Without touching her drink, the woman stubs out her cigarette and immediately lights another. She looks at her wristwatch and scowls. I order a cappuccino while she drums her lacquered nails on the tabletop. In the distance, a tall handsome man with floppy black hair is flirting with the colourfully dressed girls. The sound of their laughter makes the woman sitting next to me look up. Downing her coffee in one, she turns her back to the square while the man makes his way towards the café. Even with his hands stuffed into his pockets, he walks like a movie star.

"*Ciao Bella!*" The dark-haired man sits down next to her. Leaning forward, he makes to kiss her but the woman turns her cheek away.

Tom is nowhere to be seen. I skim the froth on my cappuccino with a spoon and cast an envious eye at the cake display. Half-heartedly I try to attract a waiter but my eye is drawn to the couple. She is pouting while the man talks. His tone pleading, he knots his hands as if in prayer – as if this woman were more Madonna than Venus.

Tom and I never argue. When I first mentioned art classes, Tom said, "You can't paint." He's always got an answer ready. It's easier to say nothing. The following week, on my afternoon off, I took a bus to the seaside. It was one of those crisp, cold sunny days. The whole beach was deserted, except for a woman exercising a horse on the sands. I sat for hours in the dunes – watching, drawing. Balancing my sketchpad on my knees, I tried to capture that animal's long grey legs, its sleek neck and tousled mane until my fingers were frozen. When I got home, I showed Tom my efforts. He said it looked like next-door's dog.

Humming something operatic under his breath, the waiter busies himself delivering mountains of spaghetti to a tour-bus party. I decide against the cake for now and cast another glance at the couple. The dark-haired man has stopped pleading. He is more animated. His voice is raised and his hands fly in all directions as if swatting an imaginary wasp. The woman's cigarettes sit on the table between them. Apparently exasperated, the man takes one from the packet and signals his order with a flick of his wrist. His pale companion points at the girls across the square. Laughing, the man shrugs his shoulders. Silently setting the drink down in front of him, the waiter scuttles off. Then with one swift deft motion the woman tilts the table, propelling hot coffee on to the man's lap. Yelling, he leaps up and tries to wipe away the stain with a napkin. Waiters nudge each other, playfully rolling their eyes to heaven – as if they're used to such outbursts. "It would never happen in England. . ."

That's what Tom would say if he could see them. When he criticised my sketch of the horse, I said nothing. Then he looked at me and said, "Oh for Heaven's sake, it's only a picture."

The woman gathers her things. Suddenly I wish I had a pencil and paper so I could catch the expression on her face. I want to fathom that look, dissect it, preserve it – have it framed on my wall so I can see it daily. Some things can't be expressed in words – that's why there's art and music. Next term I won't let Tom talk me out of those night classes.

Blonde curls trailing, the woman saunters off across the square. When she reaches the girls in bright dresses she snaps her fingers and tosses her mane. They do not retaliate. Next to this vision of Venus, they cease to look exotic. Their tanned skin and brown hair seem ordinary, their florid clothes look cheap and garish.

Reaching into his pocket, the man slams a fistful of euros down on the wet tabletop and storms off. His swagger gone, he looks foolish in his coffee-stained pants. Customers snigger openly as he limps by. I look back at the blonde woman across the piazza. She does not turn round to view the shock waves in her wake. Cool and triumphant, she disappears into the same dark street that I walked along only moments before.

"Getting fat on cake are we?"

Squinting against the sun, I look up and see Tom standing beside me. I hadn't noticed him cutting across the square.

"Well, was it worth it?" He pulls up a chair and sits down. All about us, conversations resume as if nothing has happened. People in the piazza carry on like extras in a film. Tom puts his fingers into my glass of water and scoops out an ice-cube. His forehead his damp – he swipes it with the back of his hand. Sucking on the ice, he smiles. As I slide the water over to him, the glass leaves a trail on the tabletop between us. Tom takes a mouthful, unaware that he has missed all the drama. Across the square, the girls in bright dresses are talking to a group of boys on mopeds. Their skirts ride up as they climb on to the backs of the boys' scooters and speed away. Without them the piazza seems still and calm. I am reminded of water closing over the head of a submerged diver. It's as if a video of Botticelli's painting has been played in reverse – instead of Venus rising from the foam she has slid beneath the waves, leaving no visible hint of what went before.

Tom studies the menu. "Well, was it worth it?"

I look at him quizzically.

"Getting up early to see what's its name? You know – Venus on a soap-dish. . ."

Graham Clifford

Stealing summer

He sprawls among pregnant old men
bewildered in baseball caps,
and bristled, pork-crackling wives.

Worn-out evergreens flop and nod
insects into the bright, cyan pool.

His wife swats a butterfly off her belly.
She Velcros on a tin-foil collar
to encourage sunlight up her nose,
a smudge of amber flying-powder
on the back of her hand.

The ancient, hotel moggy pads over
dozy from being black in the sun
to show off a blood-flecked starfish
twitching at the base of its question mark tail.

It's always summer here. Or at least late spring.
Daydreaming at a gull,
his gaze snags on the chalk-dust moon.
Orchids blurt livid Rorschach smears and polka dots.
A tights-coloured jelly-fish flops and folds over
and inside-out in a meek tide
that thrums the beach like it's at work
and being watched.

He barely sleeps all week,
garlic soup and frappé fermenting
along sore, demijohn innards.
But when his lids do slide closed,
his Lilo chafing the pool side's concrete lip, or
twisted into his sheets, a bleached dawn
at last seeping from the curtains,
he dreams a muffling inch of snow has settled
on date palms and hire cars.

Graham Clifford

Skinned

The lad in the cafe at the end of the pier
is so wrecked with puberty we're afraid he might forget
to breathe. He's a skinned nerve,
a child in a man-suit fumbling our tea and biscuits.
I pay with pocket-warm coins and our fingers rub.
He flicks a glance at me with eyes like bullet holes.

Poor sod. I remember the throb
in my leg bones in dinner queues at school;
how, elongating on the sofa I begged
mum to knead my calves; how
one muggy evening, a bloke stared back from the
wardrobe mirror
daring me with a frown to solve

the numbing blush, to explain
why his best friend was no longer anywhere near enough.

What I wrote

Do you remember what I wrote
on the back of my German book,
about Miss Moore, as some sort of joke?
And how she sent me to Fossey –
he had old elephant's ears
and a tin in his heart.

When I proffered the exercise book
he churched his fingers
and told me to read what I'd written
then read it again, but this time
                              slow,
so the words could hurt us both properly.

I read and he leaned back
away from me.

Graham Clifford

The Best Poem Ever Written

I write a poem that is the best. Massive.
I don't just mean long but
huge intellectually
and although it ends up as quite a few pages
it's so easy to read it's like freefalling –
but if you did have the willpower
to stop halfway through
you would find
each line was a whole other world, teeming
with genius-thoughts.
The poem makes me famous.
It's on the lips of intellectuals
and cleaners; teachers,
even pissheads because
the breweries print stanzas
on the bottom of beer bottles.
On hot, oxygen-depleted nights
I walk down city streets and hear
lines of my poem being whispered by
sticky people. On the tube,
I peek over the top of a book about me
at a man in a suit nodding off
and recognise the words he's mouthing
in his swoon.
All front pages, every day
have the entire poem, in small font –
bombings or muggings
get tucked inside.
All new books have my poem
printed as an introduction.
No one wants to be without it.
Systematically, everyone I have ever known
rings me to ask how I did it.
I say I don't know, and that's the truth.
After a year the fuss doesn't die down.
One morning I sit at my computer
and hear downstairs turn the TV on.
I put my ear to a gap in the floorboards.
It's an actor and he's reading my poem.
It's a good version, I've heard it before.
He has a Shakespearean voice
doing justice to what the introducer calls
The Best Poem Ever Written.
I listen to it all, I travel where the poem takes me
then get back in my chair
and write a better one.

Graham Clifford
What I really want to do

In the hotel I wait in a fresh suit,
the material hanging on me cold and heavy.
My palms are clammy, cheeks burn
from adrenalin. Muffled TV applause
and premiership results haunt the air.
I'm about to piss again when he arrives,
shakes my hand well then leads me
by the grinning receptionist, down thin stairs
past a Spanish argument in the kitchen
into the back room.

Through the net curtain there is a wall.
A two bar electric heater
from a Giles cartoon has baked the oxygen.
He asks me to sit. I already have
so he thanks me for coming and
thanks me for wearing a suit and I say
it's new, this morning, I'm trying it out
to see if it works and he laughs.

He asks the big one first,
What do I want to do? but he's friendly
and funny and he wants me to be frank
so I tell him, I'm lost, unsure
and he tells me my CV is intriguing, a jigsaw
with bits missing then extra bits,
snippets from another scene. And that's funny.
But what do I want to do?

He tells me about him: he loves opera.
His hands are thick and small and he's perspiring
in the receding Vs and he's fat and he's written
articles on interview techniques for IT graduates
and reviews opera. Sometimes he's in Geneva.
He has a suit on. No tie. It is Saturday.
But what do I really want to do?

I hold my hands out, palms up.
They're empty.

Sally Zigmond

A Twisted Thread

I first saw him as a black speck on the white plain; a man leading a starving horse; his eyes snow-blind, his cheeks sheened with fever. He came closer as I waited. He staggered and fell at my feet.

I took him into my tent, then slaughtered the mare. I made him drink what little blood it had. He drank it without knowing what he drank. He slept for three days. When I told him what I had done, he wept. I do not know why. It was more use dead and when we and the other women feasted on it I knew the lean days were over.

Yet, when they first saw him, they wanted to kill him. I stood before them and proclaimed him mine and they would touch him at their peril. Grins were exchanged. For it is known that I have never had a man.

So he stays, but shrinks into the shadows when they are here.

Now they are gone. Left behind are the toothless grandmothers, the children who are weaned from the breast and me.

And the man.

We sit with the fire between us. He is always cold although the dung fire burns hot. I weave and he talks.

He is a strange man. He is tall but has no body hair. His skin is pale gold and his hair is black. He speaks softly. The men of our tribe are stocky with beards and hair of flame. They swagger, bone daggers at their waists. They are hunters and tamers of horses.

"Your men are savage brutes," he says, although he has not yet seen them. "We live in cities. We have streets, laws and good government."

"I do not know those words," I say. He stands up and walks to the entrance of the tent and lifts the cloth.

I hear the hobbled horses strike the ground with their hooves. They ring like hammers on metal. The wind whistles through their tangled manes. The dogs by the fire grumble in their sleep. He drops the curtain I wove three summers ago. He returns to hug the fire. Then he laughs and picks a piece of flesh from his teeth. "To think I am living thus," he says.

Some days later, pounding hooves, jingling harnesses and shrill cries announce the return of the women once again. The raw air is slashed by the heat of fresh blood. A hog, thin but with meat enough upon its bones is dropped at my feet. The dogs that returned with the hunters greet those left behind with furious barks, jumping at each other's throats, tails thrashing like sword blades. The babies and toddlers wake in their woven cribs and howl. We all share the same hunger. Even the stranger.

As I put pots to heat on the fire. Olgatha enters. She helps me skin the beast and scrape it clean of flesh and fat. We throw the meat into the pots. Beneath her tunic, her new-born son suckles from her swollen breast. We work swiftly. I see the man watching her.

She was once Takalam's woman. But she is good to me. Soon the pig-flesh has devoured our hunger. Outside, the wind screams across the plain, kicking up a blizzard. The children ask for the tale of the Raven and the Foal, but I am shy in the presence of a stranger.

He lifts his head at my words. "In our land women do not tell tales. It is men such as I who sing their songs to the trill of the lyre."

"What do your women do?"

"They make themselves beautiful," he says. "For men."

Does he mock me? Despise my ugliness? I feel his eyes rake my misshapen jaw and twisted back and I want to cry.

He touches my hand. "I would like to hear your stories."

The other women have already left the tent and returned to theirs, scooping up the sleeping children under their arms. We are alone. I reach for my knife I use to sever the yarn and the cord that binds the newborn to their mothers. "No stranger steals the stories from our ancestors. I will not tell you."

The night passes with no word between us. The wind drops and the tent sighs and stiffens with ice. The fire burns low. I concentrate on my loom, keeping count of the warp threads, changing the colours, the twisting of the weft beneath and over the warp. Which is he and which is I?

"Where are the men?" he asks the following day.

"Away." I do not wish to think of the men.

"Why are they not here to take care of their women and children? Provide for them?"

"Women do not need men."

Just then, one of Olgatha's tall daughters enters the tent and shyly hands me a skein of thread she has spun herself. I inspect it thoroughly for knots and burrs. I find none. She goes away, her braided head tilted with pride.

"If men and women live apart, where do the young come from?"

I have to explain the simplest things. "The men come every second full moon. When they come they take away the boys who have grown beards and plant their seed within us, then leave. It is the custom."

"But what of love?" he whispers. He is a strange man.

Now the days and nights stand as equals. Soon the days will begin to nibble the tails of the night and grow longer before the nights exact their revenge, as the old tales tell us. The grass grows again. Today I freed the horses from their ropes. They careened across the plain rolling over and over, kicking up their back legs and playing the fool. They soon settle, their shaggy necks curved to crop the first sweet shoots of the season. Their tails flick. The flies are waking too and cloud their heads. The whole world is yawning. The sky is the colour of skimmed milk thawing in the bowl.

The moon is full tonight. Tonight the men will come. The children are excited, especially the boys. They squabble and the women cuff them about their ears. Those who will leave with them on the morrow strut like warlords.

I lift the entrance cloth. The sun stabs the floor and slices the body of the stranger who has just risen from his sleep. His back is to me. He lifts a bowl of mare"s milk from the fire and places it on the rug-strewn floor. He takes a piece of foal-skin, swishes it in the steaming liquid, squeezes out the excess moisture and applies it to his body. Then he dips his face in the now cool liquid and splashes it about his face before applying a sharp blade to his cheeks. I have touched this blade. It is sharp and cold beneath my finger. When he has finished he puts the used milk to one side. He has learned that we waste nothing. The children will use it to make supple the saddles and soak the read stems ready to fashion into arrow shafts.

It is strange to me, this desire to remove the signs of manhood. A beard divides the man from the boy. His people must remain as children until they die. And yet he tells me how the call to manhood is strong in his land. He tells me that when the sun blazes fiercely above their heads they engage in vigorous sports, testing each others' strength to the very limits of endurance: running, wrestling, throwing wooden spears and discs of stone.

And now he stands up and turns to face me. The shaft of sunlight ripples across his nakedness. For a moment we gaze upon each other in wonder. I now see the beauty of the clean, white, male form. He is less thin than he was when he arrived and his muscles are well-formed. I see each sinew beneath the skin. He only shaves his face and head. There is a straggle of hair on his chest and his cock stirs within a nest of black curls.

He is without his beard but a man for all that.

He binds a piece of cloth about his waist and strides from the tent on sturdy legs, passing close to me as he does. He smells of the spring sky and fresh grass. I watch him go. Slowly at first as if testing his muscles, he begins to run, picking up speed, bearing down upon the group of horses. They scatter, whinnying in alarm, tossing their heads, their hooves pounding the plain, before regrouping and continuing to graze.

I am used to solitude. But I have never felt lonely until this moment.

The other women are dressing their hair in tight braids, twisting strings of wool around them. They are laughing, showing their fine pointed teeth. They take it in turns to drag bone combs through the tangled flames of their hair.

I take no part in this but continue at my loom, thinking about the stories I will tell during the feast tonight. The stranger is returned. He squats beside me, shooting a quiverful of questions about what happens when the men come.

"What do you think happens when men meet women?" I laugh and am surprised by my own bitterness. I stand back and regard the cloth stretched across my loom. That at least is fruitful. The stranger has said much about the strange land in which he lives. There are beasts with skins of leather like the snake but walk on four legs. Their are creatures that can live in pools of water. Their skins are featherless but they fly like birds through the water, which he says is wider than the plain, which is impossible. He says horses gallop across these watery plains, wild and snarling, full white tails streaming behind them like clouds presaging a storm. Beneath them fly the water-birds in all the colours of the known world, but more dazzling, more alive.

I recreate these strange beasts and weave them into my cloth. I will tell tales of these creatures that drink nectar from heart of flowers the size of our round tents and the colour of blood. For that is what the stranger tells me. He has made my world wider and brighter. I see beyond the brown plain, further than the edges of my mind. I feel my body stretch and strengthen.

Suddenly the women leap up and the children run screaming towards the horizon.

"The men are coming," I tell him and he too rises and makes his way to the curtain and pushes it aside.

"I see nothing," he says.

"Look again," I command him as I would a child. "Do you not see the sky darken beneath the cloud of dust that rolls towards us? How in the name of our ancestors do you defend yourselves? Do you lie down and offer your necks like curs?

I know my words have stung him. I wish they had not but I am sharp because the men have come. I have never heeded their indifference to me nor longed for their fierce embraces, but today I feel bereft, jealous of the rough attention that will be denied me. My thoughts are as tangled as raw yarn and I sense something of the excitement the other women feel and thought would never be a part of me.

The stranger too is as tense as a strained bow before the arrow flies. I see a vein in his neck throb. He is right to be afraid.

The feast is over. The boys have been handed over to the care of the men and they are enjoying their first taste of fermented mare's milk. It is always a moment for laughter as they splutter and cough and then grow sleepy. The men lie with the women in their arms, slowly stroking their bodies, savouring the pleasures to come. Some couples, the eager ones, have already slipped away to other tents.

But my tent remains full. Someone mouths a tuneless song until kicked into silence. Dogs nose the rugs, seeking discarded bones and licking grease from the children's faces. Moisture glistens on the skins hanging on the walls and trickles to the floor.

One of the men calls out to me. "Old Crone! Tell us the tale of the braggart, Vostik, and how his sword was stolen as he fucked his master's wife."

"No," cries another. "I want to hear of the passion of Urmlich for the queen of the Ice."

I stand up knowing that I will have to tell them both and many more before they will let me rest.

Takalam staggers to his feet. Takalam, my twin. My womb-companion. He sways glowing in the firelight, a giant who fiery head butts against the roof. His green eyes are fixed upon the stranger, my stranger, who is looking elsewhere, gravely regarding two women who are beginning a slow, sinuous dance, weaving between the couples, placing their bare toes in the men's mouths and snatching them back before they are bitten. I should have warned him. He should not look upon them. They are Takalam's new women and Takalam is a jealous man.

We dwelled in the womb together for nine months, our bodies twisted so tightly together our mother was cut apart to give us life. Takalam was lifted out as true and strong as a mighty tree. I was peeled from around him, a weak vine, twisted and bent. Yet, we are matched. We are both proud of our skills, but he is as handsome as I am ugly. He is harsh and I am gentle. My mind is true; his is twisted. Say one word to defy him and he cuts your throat. I have seen it.

Takalam has seen. The tent falls silent, but for the snoring of the dogs and the hiss of the fire. He draws his bone-blade from his waist and points it at me.

"The cripple has not yet told us the tale of this cuckoo in our nest. Why is he here? What does he want of us?"

Sneering laughter crackles around the tent. "Does he want to steal a woman?" he jeers. "Does he know what to do with one?"

More laughter – dangerous low laughter.

"Does he wish for the wild Olgatha?" Takalam despises Olgatha because she would not give him a son. He aims a boot at her backside, almost knocking her into the fire. She snarls and retreats to the edge of the crowd. "Or this one?" He pulls a woman from the floor by her braids. "But, remember. If you take her, I will slice the head from your shoulders and feed it to the dogs!"

Thin laughter dribbles from the drunken men like piss from a frightened dog.

Takalam speaks again. "Perhaps not, eh, stranger?" Then he slaps his leather thighs and the dogs leap up barking until he roars them to silence. "Listen. I have a better idea. Let him have my sister. No-one else wants her!"

He taunts the stranger. "Do you have a sword?"

One of his lackeys takes up the cry. "It will be but a blade of winter grass, soft and withered!"

"Show us your reed-pipe and pipe us a tune!"

"If he can find it!"

I flash a warning glance at the stranger but I am too late. Takalam leaps on him, then his cousin, Gangest and more and more. Even some of the younger, sillier women crawl over him and claw at his garments, giggling over his bare legs, kissing his bare buttocks.

I peer between my fingers. I see Takalam seize the stranger by his ears and haul him to his feet, gasping and spluttering. His nose pours blood and his face is bruised. He is naked. Teeth marks scour his back, his legs, his arms.

He bears his humiliation with dignity.

But I am ashamed. Of my people and that I dwell among them.

I take the knife from my belt. I slice the warp threads from the top and bottom of my loom. I shake the cloth to life. It is the red of blood, woven with the fishes of the blue and green water, the dazzling white mares of the mighty ocean that is wider than the plains. It is strange. It is magnificent and my people gasp.

I take it to the man and with it clothe his naked and wounded body. Carefully, slowly I fasten shoulder and hip buckles from carved bone and take the girdle from my waist and tie it around his. My people watch. They know what it means. It is known that this prize should be Takalam's and therefore it is known that he is slandered and humiliated. Takalam's mouth hangs open like an old saddle-bag. I approach him boldly and take the sword from his belt and present it to the stranger.

"Leave us now," I say to the stranger. "Go home and tell your people about us. Not of Takalam. He is rabid wolf, foaming at the mouth when the moon is full. But of our land and our ways."

He nods. "You have taught me much," he says. "This garment and the giving of it tell me everything."

"Tales are tales. Only this is true." I place his hand on my heart.

The next morning when only I am awake, I stand on the plain and watch the sun rise. The dawn wind ripples through the grass and a tiny feather flutters to my feet. I take it back to my loom and weave it into a new story.

Joan Michelson

Shield

Maybe
in my last years

I will
build a house.
Maybe

I will build
and sing
in the branches

scratching
at the window.

If I don't return,
maybe you
will make

a home
in my room.
Books piled

on the shelf.
A round ceramic

lamp. Words
like moths
opening their wings.

Second Anniversary

Two years (next week, two years) from where we stopped,
I bicycle along the roads and see you
everywhere in everything, no longer
human-you, yet not ineffable

like wind, or this warm breath of mist; but root,
bulb, road-side magnolia bloom blown fat
with brown-tipped buds; and roses, pink and full,
as if no winter is, though winter was.

Sap-slowed, in leaf, this winter is; but not.
I remember nights in our worn bed,
a year perpetual with winter cold.
How then this limbo season like a tease?

How I, loosened out of disbelief,
flower as if risen up for Christmas.

Christmas Crow
(in homage to CK Williams)

Crow spread in the green scum of the pond, heavy and dark on
 Christmas morning,
his wing broken, or something keeping him lurching from side-to-side
 the few metres
until finally, he paused, his head against the black plastic lining rising
 to the rocks.

And I saw, despite his eye flickering in warning of a savage
 endurance,
the wings fold, the way a body folds into itself and slides out of the
 future,
and a kind of terror shook me as if the worst was to drown in my
 garden pond.

But he wasn't dead yet. It was barely noon. And when he rolled from
 the spread prongs
of the grass rake, gentle enough with its flexible stub ends and I,
 timidly determined,
covered him with a kitchen cloth, one wing was opening again and I
 felt uncertain.

What of the fire yet in him? What of the silence ready to break at his
 abhorrent caw?
The next day his legs – the white, scaly, translucent with claws –
 were raised against his breast
and when I lifted him, I felt the emptiness. Hard it was, but oh so
 light.

Joan Michelson

The Last Week

On the Sunday we went for coffee.
With my leg in plaster
and my crutches, I went slowly,
I told you, *Go ahead*
I met the phys-ed teacher
who does Astanga yoga
He had half an hour. Good,
I said, *Come meet Geoff.*

Next time I saw the phys-ed teacher
was the Thursday after.
I told him you were dead.
He looked at me, *But*

we just met. I said, *It happened.*
I didn't see him after that.
I heard he returned to Sydney
with a girl he met.

So we had coffee Sunday. Monday
my plaster cast came off.
We took the bus together Tuesday.
Because I stood, you snapped.

Wednesday you had your hair cut.
Of Thursday I remember
you gave your evening class a miss
and did some desk work.

Friday we were at the pool,
the three of us together.
I was still counting lengths
when you left for work.

You called out, *Enjoy your trip*,
Shopping, I groaned, *See you.*
On the Saturday we saw you.
Then we found your will

and the letter-poem *Satan*
filed in your computer.
It was time-marked two a.m.
that Friday, your death day.

Joan Michelson

Brief Bliss

I saw something rise, or something hung
above the border of the dark, and left
something swollen. It was orange. It was
yellow as a egg yolk. And a cow
was lowing. Then I smelled a stink of bull,
that bull rubbing off against the fence,

or was this nonsense drawn from my confusion
in the dawn of autumn? in the brush
of scarlet, orange, yellow-gold and brown,
oaks and elders standing where a single
school girl, waiting for a school bus, held
a roll of paper with a picture that she

might have showed me if the sky had
lightened up more quickly. As it was,
the sun did not appear for half an hour. The light
up there, now that the moon, for moon it must
have been, hung like the egg-yolk sun
too early in the dawn, had disappeared,

the sky was simply pale as if washed out,
and in that Pale of Sky although the animals
(and I) were all awake, the wind lay down
and it was still as if the seasons, autumn,
winter, spring, and summer too, or time,
was crushed like leaves inside a burlap sack

and dropped beyond the ridge of forest road
and so in grey like bliss outside of hours
I strolled along that road for half an hour
until above a hill, light rose. It was
the sun. And at that stroke of blinding which I
clocked, a winter wind reared up and bit.

Tom Bryan

Sister of the Sun

No life can be contained in a shoe box. But this shoe box is different. The joy and pain it contains can only be known if the rest of its story is known, even if forgetting would be less painful.

***

We were very different immigrants, Sun Sister and myself. I had come to America to study linguistics at the State University, on the way to wanting to be a poet. Scotland via Canada. Sun Sister had come from an "emerging" African nation to study. She spoke her own tongue and some other African languages, as well as French and German. We sat next to each other in our Introductory Linguistics class. She spoke first. "Alistair, yours is a fun name to say. My own name is so difficult for Westerners. *Alayla* is the closest you might come. It means The Sister of the Sun." So, *Sun Sister* she always was. Myself, short and stocky, fair, freckled. Alayla, tall, stunningly black, with high cheekbones and hair swept up and back.

I remember that first day so well. After class, we walked out into the September sun, through the arboretum. The maple trees ablaze, the last butterflies of the year resting on the limestone walls; crickets and grasshoppers buzzing. "Well, Alistair (she said it with more syllables somehow, eyes full of laughter) "you know many westerners think we Africans wear straw skirts and live in straw huts, and go without shoes. Let me show you a photograph." The photo showed Alayla, in grass skirt, in a straw hut. The entire family was without shoes. She laughed and her cheekbones danced with that laughter. And I who know nothing of girls or women (I am one of five boys) thought I was in love. She took my hand that day and we walked and talked until darkness came, when I walked her home to her hall of residence.

She was an outstanding student. Her essays and exams were always top of the class, while I struggled, especially with language theory. Sometimes I watched her from the corner of my eye. Her own face shifting from serious to happy, her long body relaxed in a floral skirt. Yet she made few friends and seemed to like my company, and often encouraged me to write poetry. I should say from the start in two full years we were never lovers, only kissing innocently sometimes and holding hands, but we were inseparable.

My uncle farmed nearby and he welcomed us both into his big family, He had four sons and three daughters and Alayla soon felt at home there, reading stories to the children. "Alayla do they have lions where you live? Have you ever seen a giraffe? Or a crocodile?"

She would flash her teeth and growl. "I have not seen a lion, I AM ONE" and chase the wee ones around the room.

Our first year together was like a childhood dream. In autumn, we rode bikes out into the country on weekends, gathering persimmons,

wild apples or hickory nuts, taking long walks through forests of maple and yellow poplar, leaves crisp underfoot. She was keen to have photos of everything:
  Alayla buying pumpkins at a roadside stall.
  Alayla eating persimmon pudding.
  Alayla dancing around a bluegrass fiddler.
  Alayla hanging upside down from a maple tree.
  Alayla roasting corn on an open fire.
  Alayla pitching horseshoes.
Winter brought sled rides down the campus hills, holding on to each other, Alayla shrieking and laughing in the snow, her first experience of it. Building snowmen, then banging into them until they fell to pieces, then patiently rebuilding them again Then we would go to the Union for coffee or hot chocolate or sometimes back to her hall for tea. I stayed with my uncle five miles away, driving into class each day, often following the snow plough into town.
  Sister of the Sun never talked about herself or her family. Instead, she often asked about mine: "Your mother, what was she like?"
  I laughed in reply. "Alayla, just look at me. Red and freckled. She was five feet tall. No woman of her era was allowed to be taller than five feet. A Scotswoman through and through. *Awa an bile yer heid. Haud yer weesht. Ah'll skelp yer lugs. That's me, awa fer thi messages.* Her only brother came from Scotland to marry a Red Cross nurse he met in the war so I've come to stay with them until my course is finished. My mother died of cancer at the age of 45 so me and my four brothers scattered, in Canada and America." Alayla took my hand. "Family, it is all we are. It is what we are." That was the Sister of the Sun. We took a night walk in the snow, the ice glinting from the tree branches, snow piled against the walls, stars sparkling, her hand tight in mine. Now and then, snow fell from the boughs, leaving a trail of muted notes in the dark. Her cold breath clouded around her dark face.
  "My own land – Alistair – it is painful. So full of promise and hope, especially after our independence. Now, it is just tribal loyalties bubbling to the surface. My own father is a newspaper editor who was able to criticise the previous regime but after promises of liberal reform and tolerance, I think this new government will go the same way as the previous one. My father is angry at the failed promises and feels he can only carry on with his criticisms. He and many others feel betrayed and cheated by the current government. He's very proud of his native land but he also feels he must tell the rest of the world what is going on. But the government is very sly. Our leader is outwardly calm and respectable, presenting a good face to the West but secretly, he is watching to see who he has to fear. Already he has offered my father a lucrative government job on condition he quits editing the paper. One by one, he is trying to buy off all his potential critics but those refusing his largess will be marked men and women, especially if they are not

of his tribe or language. That is why I am so interested in linguistics. In our country, it can be a matter of survival. Our native language marks you for life, for good or bad."

Her hand gripped mine even more tightly. The glint of a street light showed the tears streaming down her eyes. We walked on in the snow, it rustling soft on her coat, her shoulders hunched, making her seem so small and vulnerable, despite her great height.

Alayla went to Paris for Christmas and all her family came from various countries to be there. I spent my own Christmas with my nieces and nephews scampering over each other to open presents. I read them stories and played with their new toys, all the while thinking about the Sister of the Sun, so far away on this cold winter's day. It snowed until well past New Year. When she returned, she told me her father was not able to leave Africa to come to Paris. She never said why. The winter went slowly. Snow, deep and lingering, never melted in the sub-freezing temperatures. Weekdays we studied together, curled up on her sofa, her legs tucked under mine, us both sipping tea. Weekends took us to my uncle's farm or for long walks along the frozen river. Alayla's eyes missed nothing, as though she might not be here again, might not remember. Always, she encouraged me to write, to record everything. She pretended to chastise me once. "You are a lazy poet. You should be writing all the time, surrounded by piles of poetry. In my country, poets are revered because they are often in trouble with the authorities, who know how much damage a good poem can do. So write, lazy man, write. Hey you, tell me what you see right now."

Alayla is sitting on a stump under a bare persimmon tree. The river is grey behind her, frozen and still. She is grinning. Her whole body is grinning. She wears a woollen hat with ear flaps, her dark hair springing out wildly. She is eating a piece of chocolate. Against all the grey, she is the only living colour, black against the melting snow. Behind her, dark snow clouds were rolling in over the forest and fields of stubble.

Spring came suddenly. The creeks filled with rushing snowmelt, fat robins hopped on the lawns for worms, everything thawing and rushing, flowers, grass and blossoms. The forests thickened with colour. Warm days brought out butterflies: mourning cloaks, skippers and tiger swallowtails. Alayla was always most alive and most alert in the forests and the deeper into the forest the more she laughed and talked. We were looking for morel mushrooms, their fusty strong smell so overpowering among the pines. We were careful to look out for copperheads sunning themselves after a hard winter, these snakes the colour of a new penny. Alayla alert, so purposeful, gathering mushrooms which we later coated in egg and cornmeal, frying them, feeding them to one another. Alayla in jeans, muscled like a panther, white cotton shirt, brown eyes peeking under her errant hair, smiling, eyebrows raised for mischief. "Some of the African brothers don't like me spending so much time with a white boy but I told them to mind their own business. They do not understand. They will never understand. That kind of thinking is tearing my own country apart." I realised then how special, how different this Sun Sister was. She went back to Africa that first summer. I drove her to the local airport for a quick flight to the big airport. She hugged me so tightly, I felt every curve of her and she kissed me quickly and walked to the plane, never looking back.

My own summer passed slowly. I helped my uncle with the hay, rising at five in the morning, hoping for a strong morning sun to dry the bales, mindful of the weight of them when wet. We drank cold water, eating sandwiches in the shade, the sun already bleaching my hair. Bales of sweet grass, timothy or clover, stacked on the flatbed, then loaded in the barn. I was exhausted at night, hardly able to eat my aunt's dinner of fried chicken with sweet corn and cornbread. If I couldn't sleep, I always thought of Alayla, so strange to me, her life so different and so far away. I puzzled over her friendship with me. Alongside her I felt so gauche and self-conscious yet she herself did nothing to make me feel that way. She was always interested in my life, in my poetry, in my uncle and aunt, my nieces and nephews. Yet she maintained that quiet aloofness, that need not to be hurt. My heart was pounding the day I fetched her at the airport in late summer. She wore white cotton. Her hair was cut differently, showing off her cheekbones and big eyes even more but something was gone, a light, a shining. That light never came back.

We walked under the trees as we did before, hand in hand. If anything, Alayla clung even harder, wrapped into me even more, but was even more silent. One evening, she never stopped crying.

"My father is being threatened now by the very regime he had such faith in. They want him to stop writing for the newspaper. Oh, the pressure is enormous. Promises of a new house, foreign holidays, a job with government public relations. He wants to emigrate now, maybe even come here but that would also be difficult. He has lived there all his life and is proud of his new state. He is a patriot in the good sense."

I sensed her desperation in the second year. She studied less, was more insistent on long walks.

Alayla, Sister of the Sun is sitting in the sun, on a big pile of raked maple leaves. There is a Golden Rain Tree behind her. The limestone walls and buildings are glistening. She broods. She doesn't know I have photographed her. Her lean body is in the picture but her mind is thousands of miles away. Sometimes, Alayla would disappear for days at a time, missing classes. Nobody in her hall knew where she was. She would come back, take my hand in hers and walk, saying nothing, squeezing my hand. The day was a soft autumn day at the farm, pigs fed, barn checked, tractors and equipment cleaned and put away. Indian Summer, a lazy Saturday. People would be at the football game, maybe just sitting on their porches listening to crickets and grasshoppers sawing away. My uncle was pitching horseshoes around the back, the clang of a ringer, children shouting, farm dogs barking. I took a long shower and drove into town, to Alayla's. The town was deserted, everyone doing something somewhere else, leaves rustling under the maples lining every street, streets Alayla and I had walked hand-in-hand in every season, in wind, snow and rain. She wasn't in her hall of residence but Theresa, from the Cameroons, gave me a note from Alayla:

Dear Alistair,

Don't worry, I will be back. I had to go home. There was bad news about my father. If anything happens to me Theresa will give you a shoe box. You are a poet, you will know what to do with it if you read what is written there. I want to thank you for being my friend and for being so kind to me. Please do not worry. I would like to come back and maybe we can be more than friends for I am thinking more about love now. Maybe I am ready for this but please do not worry about me. My father is a brave man and no harm will come to him.

Love, Sister of the Sun

***

The shoe box accuses me. It lives under my bed where it has been for three years. Alayla's country is being torn apart by tribal and civil war. Alayla's father simply disappeared and I later heard she and her sister were killed in an overturned taxi, a week after I was given her note.

I never finished the course. I haven't written a poem since then either. I work on my uncle's farm. I plant and cut corn in season, help with the hay in summer. Sometimes, on a warm summer night, while my aunt and uncle and all their children sleep, I slip out onto the porch and watch the fireflies light up the cornfields, listen to the katydids and crickets, watch the big, soft-bodied silk moths alight on the screen, leaving their coloured wing dust there. I think of the lives in that box – important letters, addresses, scribbled notes, even two love poems from Alayla, maybe to me but I will now never know for sure. I know my life will not rest until I can read everything in the box and make it come to life again. Many of the letters are to Alayla's father. Some are from the government. They may be evidence one day against a regime that probably murdered him for writing the truth. So a shoe box comes to me, on a quiet farm and countryside thousands of miles away from all that pain and strife. I could burn it and run from those memories. I could try to forget those cheekbones, those strong fingers wrapped around mine. But I know when I go into that box, I will resurrect those lives, will feel those long strong fingers curve around me again. So far, it is difficult to watch the sun climb up from behind the poplars and maples but I will have to look directly at the rising sun one day. Instead of blinding me it will give me all the light I need to see. Then as a poet, I can open the box and tell the whole world what is there.

Derek Adams

Wreckers

It's so quiet now, as I lie
waiting for sleep to come,
I can hear the last train from London
cross the distant fields
and the metronome
tick-tick of rope against mast,
on the flood tide.

When, whirring like a super 8 projector,
from out of the moonless sky, a helicopter
its searchlight a child's torch
zigzagging the River Crouch,
along the creeks it plays
hide and seeking lightless boats,
a cabin cruiser with a cargo
of untaxed smokes
or a fishing boat from Amsterdam,
with a stow of skunk or E's or crack.

As the sound of the rotor blades fade
I remember that time, flying back
from the Thistle rig to Aberdeen,
when the Chinook's pilot took us low
over the Orkneys, to gaze
at the dark hulks breaking
the grey water of Scapa Flow.

Icarus in the 21st Century

Once dreamt of touching the stars,
now falling through the sky
burning with the beauty
of a meteorite shower.

Mission control turns blue, silent seconds –
stretch timeless towards eternity,
then like a wolf at the moon
Houston lets out a howl.

Derek Adams

A Century ago

What did they imagine, the Wright brothers,
out there at Kitty Hawk, that day,
after the Flyer left the ground for the first time.
When Orville and Wilbur
stood arms around each other
laughing and shouting,
did their thoughts soar:
to the other side of the clouds
or crossing oceans, mountains,
to a man standing on the moon, even
or how about dust
settling on rubble in Coventry
or Dresden or New York.
What would they have made
of the crew of the Enola Gay
looking back at the cloud
above Hiroshima,
or a world where
any second of the day or night
thousands of people are up in the air,
where there are so many planes
that there is not room
for them to be all on the ground
at the same time,
of an A-10 tankbuster opening fire over southern Iraq,
or a grey runway with one C-17 aircraft
its cargo being unloaded
draped in a flag of red, white and blue.

Kite

Why is it that we hold onto
this twine so tightly?
Tugging, the distant coloured kite,
that exotic dancer, gets smaller.

You pay out the line until
the kite seems just a memory,
the twine bites into your fingers
and all that's left is to let go.

Derek Adams
Prey

Hovering hawklike;
stone still and talon sharp.

      High

above my heart.

Shivering, shaking,
stopped in my tracks.
Petrified by your piercing eyes,
held in the strength of your shadow.
Prey
I wait while you

      drop

      down

      from

      the

      sky

to tear, my life to shreds.

Tania Casselle

Like Getting Caught in the Rain

Claire picked up the phone on the fourth ring.
"Can I speak with Hugh Johnson, please?" A man. Gentle tenor. Probably quite short, thought Claire.
"He's in the wardrobe," she replied.
"I'm sorry?"
"Hugh is in the wardrobe. Can I take a message?"
"What's he doing in the wardrobe?"
Claire glanced around the bedroom. The late afternoon sun seeped through the blinds, turning the light a soft liquid green, like being inside a bottle of Vinho Verde.
"Sitting on the floor, I should imagine."
"But, why?"
"I don't think there's anywhere else to sit," she offered. "It's not a very large wardrobe."
"But why don't you let him out?"
"Well, he's locked it quite firmly."
A short pause.
"Who am I talking to?" His voice was on the reedy side of tenor. Beard, decided Claire. Reddish brown beard like a fox tail.
"This is his wife."
"Ah. What I mean to say Mrs Johnson . . ."
"Ms Lynch."
". . . what I mean to say, Ms Lynch, is why is he in the wardrobe in the first place?"
"That's a good question," she mused. "I wouldn't have chosen it. The rails are rather low and between all his golf clubs on one side and my winter coats on the other, there isn't much room left in the middle. And the light bulb hasn't worked for months. Can I take your number and ask him to call you back? When he comes out of the wardrobe?"

Hugh had always been too weighed down by details. Claire had realized this on their honeymoon, when he'd joined her on a sun bed at the lip of the ocean, nothing but turquoise in sight, clear out to the horizon, with more turquoise wrapping back overhead, pierced by a high white sun. Hugh smiled at her as she lay in her new bikini, holding her book at an uncomfortable angle so the fat on the back of her arms didn't flap down, like sheets hanging in the breeze.
"Alright?" He patted her thigh. Then he took out a stack of postcards, and some sheets of pre-typed address labels, probably forty of each, and spent the entire morning selecting which scene to send to which friend, peeling the labels off one by one. He wrote a careful message on every card, blue Bic, left-handed. His arm moved like a crab, everything propelling in the wrong direction but somehow ending

up in the right place. Finally he tucked the empty sheets of waxed paper that had held the address labels under the leg of the sun bed so they wouldn't blow away, extracted forty stamps from his wallet and stuck them square as flags on each card.

It wasn't the fact that he was left-handed that surprised Claire. Of course she'd noticed that before. It had caused quite a confusion of hands in the wedding ceremony, at the part where the couple exchange rings. Hugh tried to slip the ring on her left hand with his left hand without turning too far away from the minister and appearing rude. Why couldn't he just use his right hand for once? Claire had complained silently, smiling her bride's smile. Why did he have to complicate things? He'd almost sprained his wrist, until finally she'd held out her hand, like a dog begging for a bone, so he could get a better angle on it.

No, it wasn't the fact that he was left-handed that surprised her. Even before the ring incident, she'd known it. You'd have to be fairly naïve not to realize such a thing before you agreed to marry someone, thought Claire. It had been obvious from their first meeting. He'd written his home contact details on the back of a business card, crushed up beside her on an airport bench, his briefcase a makeshift desk, his left elbow prodding rhythmically into her arm as he formed slow, sloping figures.

"You're left-handed," she observed, and leaned back a couple of inches before he started a new line and his elbow completed its trajectory towards her breast.

"Yes," he grinned ruefully. "Not superstitious, are you?"

The trouble with being so obsessed with detail, in Claire's view, was that it was like being caught in a sudden heavy rain. You didn't know whether to run for shelter, put up an umbrella, hail a taxi, or just resign yourself to getting wet. She used this analogy frequently with Hugh, and each time he just stared at her. Once, he'd replied "But it doesn't really matter which one you choose, you just pick one and do it."

"Exactly!" triumphed Claire, so Hugh had never bothered answering her again.

"You knew I was left-handed from the first time we met! I never tried to hide it!"

Hugh's last words before he slipped into the wardrobe puzzled Claire. He'd pulled the tiny key from the lock on the outside of the wardrobe door – with his left hand, Claire noted, almost defiantly with his left hand – and slammed the door behind him, then she heard the key turn. He wasn't the door-slamming type, she pondered. Even when she had dinner with her ex, Frank, and came home at half past one in the morning, slightly the worse for wear after five vodka martinis, and reported that Frank had started a horse stud operation in Hampshire and been on breakfast TV twice. Even then Hugh hadn't slammed any doors.

"Horse stud, eh?" he'd asked, stacking up a pile of photos from their weekend break in Germany that he'd spent the evening captioning and cataloguing. "Good for him." He kissed Claire on the cheek. "I think you need a cup of coffee my sweetheart. Can you remember how you spell Düsseldorf? Is it two S's or two L's?"

That was the thing about not living with someone before you married them. No matter how many weekends in country bed and breakfasts, no matter how many overnight stays and early morning rushes to work, disentangling clothes from the bed posts and jostling for the bathroom, deciding who would pick up the pizza and who would drop off the dry cleaning – all those things that were supposed to inform you about a person's secret habits and hidden vices, supposed to teach you tolerance and how to think of 'we' instead of 'I' – the point was that none of it counted until you actually lived with someone. Moreover, as Claire had always argued, until you were actually married and there were no more outs, no options to leave, no easy midnight departures with a suitcase and a sad but clean goodbye, until then you couldn't really know what someone was like at all. She had used this logic as a hypothesis to support marriage against cohabitation, but within two weeks of the wedding she realized there was a reason why people lived together first. Claire couldn't find any means to adapt her argument in the light of her new understanding without admitting she had been wrong in the first place, so she just kept very quiet.

It wasn't only the pre-typed address labels and the way Hugh insisted on using the eggs in date order, and you couldn't complain about a husband who turned himself inside out in order to avoid offending people. People just called that sensitive, which was held to be a good thing in a man. Her unmarried friends looked at her vacantly when Claire announced, a month into marriage, that she was keeping her maiden name.

"Hugh said that was fine by him," she snapped, "as long as we make sure the authorities have it on record. He spent the whole evening printing out letters to the bank, the investment people, the pension and insurance companies. I had to co-sign every damn one of them so we would have a record of proof in case of what he calls 'an emergency'."

There was a silence while her friends took protracted sips at their Chardonnay.

"You know that barrister I dated last summer?" asked Penny, at last. "He said he would personally strangle any wife of his who refused to take his family name." She bit the end off a stick of celery and nodded ominously, her bleached blonde ponytail bobbing like an exclamation point. "That's when *I* decided to bow out."

Claire didn't think it could just be the fact that he was left-handed that sent Hugh into the wardrobe. He'd never seemed unhappy about his difference, and she couldn't remember mentioning it at all after that first meeting at Gatwick. She'd kept his business card for six weeks before calling him, and then been shocked at the shiver in her hips when she heard his voice on the answermachine. The first time they spoke directly on the phone, fifty minutes of testing questions disguised as everyday conversation, each one passing the simple prerequisites and then advancing to the more sophisticated screening, she sat on a vinyl-covered stool at her kitchen counter, squirming and wriggling until her skirt rode up over her thighs and her bare skin stuck to the seat.

They arranged to see a film the following Friday. Hugh said he'd call her back when he'd found out what was playing. At the time she thought he meant just that, although a persistent nagging in a distant cave of her mind wondered if she would ever hear from him again. After she married him, Claire realized that Hugh had probably spent days weighing up the critics, comparing reviews in the papers and on the Internet, before selecting the romantic drama he'd eventually called back to suggest.

"It's French," he said. "So you have to be OK with subtitles. But the director won the Prix de . . ." here he stumbled over a long word, making Claire worried that he was choking before she'd had a chance to see his clear grey eyes again. "And you were eating a croissant at the airport, so I guessed you were probably open to foreign stuff."

"Sounds great," said Claire, relieved.

"They say it's very romantic." Hugh paused, "so I couldn't imagine anyone better to see it with."

The estate agent had called it a walk-in wardrobe when Hugh and Claire bought the house. Claire remembered biting her lip, tempted to challenge the man with the too-white teeth and the too-big clipboard to actually try walking into it himself. Obviously he was right, she conceded now. You could walk into it. You could walk right into it and lock the door behind you and stay in there for half a day without suffocating. She assumed Hugh hadn't suffocated. He hadn't responded to her for several hours, so she couldn't be sure, but Claire knew Hugh when he was unhappy. He just closed down. Sometimes she'd find him sitting at his desk, motionless as a tropical fish in a bowl, so you think the fish is dead, hanging in the weight of water. But at the very moment you decide to scoop it out with a cup, it flashes its tail and darts to the surface in search of food.

"What are you doing?" she'd ask, disconcerted by Hugh's lack of habitual industry.

"Just watching the clock," he'd reply, not shifting his eyes from the second hand. "It's very soothing. You should try it."

"Jeff Carlton called you," Claire shouted through the wardrobe door. "He said it was about the trip to Birmingham. He's sorry to call at the weekend but it's urgent. Does he have a beard?"
No reply. Claire inspected the message in her hand as if it might offer further clues. "I have his number here. I'll pass the phone in if you'll open the door a crack?"
The fake mahogany panelling remained resolutely closed. Claire picked at the tinny gilt hinge with her fingernail.

She'd told Hugh to change the light bulb in there three times. Each time he'd nodded and said it was on his list of things to do, but the list was as long as his left arm and changing the bulb in the wardrobe had never yet risen to first place.
"Why don't you pass half this stuff to your secretary?" Claire had asked him, running her eye down the inventory of numbered details. "If you lived to a hundred you could never finish all this."
"Can't trust anyone else to do it right," Hugh answered, his eyes fixed on the clock.

Claire found a new bulb in the kitchen. She tore off the white cardboard wrapper and marched upstairs.
"Here's a light bulb for you, Hughie," she called. "I'm going to lay it down outside the wardrobe door and then I'm going to back out of the room. No tricks."
She waited in the hall for fifteen minutes before she heard the click of the key.
"Hugh!" Claire lunged into the bedroom, just in time to see his left hand, clutched around the bulb, disappear into the wardrobe like a startled mouse.
"Oh, dammit Hugh! Come OUT will you? This is ridiculous."
A thin vertical strip of yellow light appeared between the doors.
"OK," said Claire. "I'll cross that one off your list, shall I?"

When the phone rang again, Claire was sleeping. She sat up, fully clothed in the darkness, and glanced towards the wardrobe. The doors were still shut, the light now off. The alarm clock glowed red. 8:23 pm.
She grabbed around for the phone. "Yes?"
"Is Hugh Johnson there?"
"I gave him your message," she sighed. "He's not come out yet."
"Do you think he might need a doctor?"
"A doctor?" Claire shook her head impatiently. "It's not a sickness to be left-handed you know. There's thousands of people like it. They even make special scissors."
"I mean there's obviously something very wrong, Ms Lintz."
"Lynch."
"He obviously needs help. And you sound exhausted."

Claire reached over to switch on the bedside lamp. From the wardrobe she heard a low snore, a body shifting, then the muffled clatter of golf clubs.

"It's just all the details, Mr Carlton," she explained. "It's like getting caught in the rain."

Elzabeth Tate

Retreat

silence
of all things
is open to
interpretation
has a capacity
to soothe
or corrode it
can be filled
with possibilities
or empty of
meaning.
neglectful
abandoned
heavy with
implication
doubt.
busy bustling
with imperatives
or just
a heavy heart
beating
a tattoo
against a wall of
silence
invisible and
impenetrable.

In the MeanTime

I hold my breath
I shave my head
I don armour
I go to war
I apply heat
I hang fire
I trawl the depths
I try on masks
I polish pebbles
I chew grit
I walk sideways
I cut swathes
I consult oracles

Elzabeth Tate

I mark graves
       in order to stay alive
       in the meantime.

Winter Landscape

The sky is made of marbled strips
in impossible colours
opalescent.
the air crisp and
dusted blueish.
the ground under my feet
pock-marked and
unrelenting
it's difficult to walk with ease.
familiar routes
rendered rigid overnight
a complex tracery of hooves
to and from the meadow
not much grazing here
just a change of situation.
days are short
and numbered now.
salt on frost
glaucous
a collision of heads at tea-time
teeth on bone
a handful of blood
thin and bright.
salt in water
tepid
locates the cut
on paper
unframed
a pocket monoprint.

Relic

In the crawl space
between
your ego
and the cellar
I found a heart

wrapped in a sack
covered in
callouses
and studded with what
looked like lead
bright-cut and cross-
patterned.
twin chambers
pumped impulsively
carrying colours
intense in motion
and redolent of
treasures glimpsed in
passing
arranged symmetrically for
people with time to kill.
a detached relic –
booty –
in the name of love.
spin-offs
from the power station
overhead keep
this swag ticking
charged
hidden from view
and its breathless owner.

Netted

duped
by amplification
and imitation.
each one
I imagine
leaves a stain
on the air
a burn in the sheet
a mote
in the sky
as it hurtles
groundward
altrical
hopeful.
a misted stimulus

Elzabeth Tate

initiates
and instigates.
a compulsive
curtain call
live-wired and
black-spotted
beware the song
of the gourmet.

Chris Turner

Elizabeth French's Irrational Fear of Chocolate

In all her life there had never been a moment when Elizabeth French had not been terrified of chocolate. The comforting, smooth, addictive treat that brought a sense of indulgence and well-being to most of her friends brought only fear and panic to Elizabeth. Even as a very small child the mere sight of a chocolate bar sent her into a screaming fit that might last for hours, puzzling parents and doctors alike, who could offer no resolution to the problem other than to recommend that child and chocolate be kept well apart.

It soon became apparent that it was not only the sight of chocolate that disturbed her. When well-meaning Aunt Helen famously remarked to four-year-old Elizabeth "Your mother must have been frightened by a Smartie at some time," it had taken the rest of the family half a day to calm Elizabeth, and all but ruined the wedding at which Elizabeth was intended to be a bridesmaid.

For her school-friends the playground proved to be a minefield of chocolate indulgence. While they stuffed their faces with chocolate biscuits, bars and rolls, Elizabeth hid herself away and read a book in order to take her mind to another place, a place devoid of chocolate and all its derivatives.

In the eventuality that the other children craved entertainment rather than chocolate it was not unusual for some or all of them to corner the unfortunate Elizabeth and taunt her with Wagon Wheels, Kit Kats and Fruit and Nut bars until she lay a screaming, shivering wreck at their feet and in need of rescue by some informed teacher or attendant.

Indeed it had occasionally happened that new or stand-in teachers had not been informed of little miss French's condition and more than one had been guilty of innocently offering a tin of chocolate confection round the class (usually in an effort to buy silence or co-operation), only to watch in horror as one of their flock ran screaming and sobbing from the classroom, with the explanation by the other children that, "It's only Elizabeth French Miss, she's frightened of chocolate," as though it were the most normal thing in the world.

Which to Elizabeth it was! As normal as breathing or singing or skipping or, she reasoned with herself, as other children's fear of the dark or snakes or spiders like Maria Clarke.

Maria had been a particularly obnoxious thorn in Elizabeth's side; exposing her weakness at every available opportunity; usually for the gratification of a cruel prepubescent audience which delighted in Elizabeth's obvious distress when she opened her desk to find a Walnut Whip sitting atop her school-books, or a Flake wrapper secured about her pen or pencil.

In her efforts to cope with a chocolate-riddled world and the sadistic monsters inhabiting it Elizabeth learned to fight back, to observe her tormentors, seek out their personal weaknesses and then strike, as she did with Maria Clarke upon discovering her terror of spiders.

For a week Elizabeth collected every spider she could find. She searched hedges and bushes, lawns and paths. The furthest recesses of the garage and the dark corners of the cupboard under the stairs, where her father kept his golf clubs and some rather odd magazines.

She collected and stored them in a cardboard box. She had fat spiders and thin spiders, smooth spiders and hairy spiders, spiders with small bodies and long legs, spiders with large bodies and small legs and one enormous garden spider with a huge body, huge legs and a white cross on its back.

Once she had collected enough of the spiders she took them to school and, while the other pupils were in assembly, emptied the contents of her box into Maria Clarke's desk, taking good care to squish the big fat garden spider onto Maria's cheese and pickle sandwich for good measure.

This done she took the box to the waste bins at the rear of the school and ripped it into small pieces before disposing of it. She then returned late for the first lesson, with an apology for her tardiness and a class-full of witnesses who would swear that of all the children in the class, Elizabeth French was the only one who could not have caused Maria Clarke to become hysterical with fear that day.

As Elizabeth progressed through the chain of schools and colleges that would complete her education she learned not to advertise her fears and, should she slip and be discovered, fight the bullies on their own terms. Everyone, she reasoned, had fears and her own fear of chocolate was no different than another person's fear of dogs; except it was a lot easier for a person to avoid a dog than it was for Elizabeth to avoid sight or scent of foodstuffs that did not contain cocoa solids in one form or another.

She observed that the people with whom she interacted on a daily basis, her workmates and social friends, were veritable slaves to chocolate; even the seasons of the year were marked by it. Easter saw it moulded into huge, foil-wrapped eggs that were in turn filled with smaller foil-wrapped chocolates and candies, its brown sticky constituents plastered round the mouths and fingers of its tiny addicts.

Summer saw it coated over ice cream and mounted upon sticks, or pushed as a flake into some vanilla ice filled cornet, to be licked and nibbled in full and obscene view of others.

Autumn and winter saw it sprinkled upon large mugs of frothy coffee or, Elizabeth gagged at the very thought, consumed as a hot drink in its own right, while Christmas saw it pressed into religious figures in advent calendars or suspended from Christmas trees, in net bags, as gold-wrapped chocolate coins.

There was no escaping the stuff. It was baked into biscuits, studded into muffins, entombed in a brioche or drizzled over Danish pastries. It was folded into sponge cakes, grated onto trifles, melted and poured onto desserts and added to coffee as a liqueur. People drank it, sucked it, licked it and chewed it. They ate it studded with nuts or fruit or flavoured with ginger and rum.

Some bathed in its essence, some bought it as a perfume and some spread it over their partner's bodies as a precursor to the sexual act, the thought of which actually made Elizabeth vomit.

Chocolate and its all-pervading influence controlled Elizabeth's life to the extent that even the most simple of everyday tasks had to be planned with military precision.

When she eventually left home, against her parent's advice, though much to their relief, Elizabeth needed to organise her routine in order to compensate for her irrational fear. Her weekly trip to the supermarket had to be planned so that she avoided the confectionery aisle, which meant the cheese and onion crisps she so liked had to be bought from the corner shop, the one where the sweets and chocolates were not visible when she stood by the till.

Back in the supermarket she had resigned herself to buying wholemeal bread because the white bread was next to the croissants and brioches, some of them sporting chocolate, some of them reeking of the stuff.

Easter and Christmas saw her supermarket shopping curtailed and she did most of her weekly shop at the Asian food store where they sold very little chocolate and much cheaper food but was much further from her apartment.

She chose her clothing from the many catalogues that plopped through her letterbox over the course of the average year; frightened to enter a dress shop or an apartment store for fear of coming face to face with a chocolate brown blouse or sweater, for by now the very colour itself reduced Elizabeth to a cold sweat and a pounding heart and she had to flee the place as though pursued by the hounds of hell.

By the time that she was twenty-three Elizabeth had confined herself pretty much to her apartment, doing tele-sales for a nation-wide double-glazing firm, ordering meals and shopping by phone, eschewing a social life and having a pretty miserable time.

She avoided the colour brown, watched only the BBC because it showed no advertisements, read food wrappers to ensure there were no traces of chocolate in anything she ever ate and turned down a holiday she won in a magazine because its destination was Salzburg and she knew its streets were studded with chocolate shops and emporia.

Elizabeth now inhabited two worlds, one within the other; a small, chocolate-free world bounded by people and places she considered safe and a huge, hostile, dangerous world laced through with the sickly sweet confection that incessantly nibbled at the edges of her safety and her sanity.

It was on the eve of her twenty-fourth birthday, during an edition of *The Sky at Night* that Elizabeth actually contemplated suicide. Patrick Moore had introduced the words Mars and Galaxy into the same sentence resulting in her spending the next two hours retching into the toilet bowl. When she later took stock of her life she emptied her tranquillisers onto the bed beside her intending to take them all; except her doctor had changed her prescription that very day and she gazed down upon sixty small, chocolate-brown tablets. Sufficient reason for her not to swallow a single one!

The very next day Elizabeth French decided to seek professional help. Not that it was the first time she had seen someone about her problem. She had seen the school psychologist from the very onset of her classroom problems but to no avail. The very mention of the word 'chocolate' made her faint and from the psychologist's viewpoint it was nigh impossible to help a child when he could not even mention the root cause of her phobia.

"A fear of chocolate," was his final diagnosis, "to which exposure, or its packaging or even the word itself, engenders an irrational, hysterical and sometimes violent response more likely to cause danger to Elizabeth herself than to others." But that was then. The in-between years had been bearable with a certain amount of environmental management. Though her choice of friends, of venues, of social arrangements had made her seem manipulative and 'strange' to the point where she found herself increasingly alone and prey to her fears.

But now she was determined to regain her life. She would not become a prisoner to chocolate, she would fight back in any way that she could and her opening salvo was to make an appointment with a phobia counsellor.

Mr Fellows held his clinic at the local hospital. He was an intense and patient man who had many questions for Elizabeth. Was she, he enquired, not so much afraid of chocolate per-se than in the effects chocolate might have upon her body? She was, after all, slim and attractive and he could well imagine the fear that could come from being addicted to chocolate and becoming what she might consider 'unattractive.'

Elizabeth answered that this was not the case, though she secretly mourned for several of her acquaintances who could not resist the stuff and had piled on the pounds because of it, one of them becoming grossly overweight. But no, Elizabeth was not afraid of the consequences of eating chocolate, simply of the chocolate itself.

Further questions elicited nothing other than Elizabeth's conviction that she should never come into contact with chocolate. She realised that it was an irrational concept, she could offer no logical reason for her belief and there was no medical evidence of a childhood allergy that might cause anaphylaxis; for she had never in her life allowed chocolate anywhere near her, a fact to which her parents could well attest.

"What are you so afraid of? What can – you know what – do to you to make you so afraid?" The counsellor eventually asked the questions that Elizabeth had been asked so many times before.

Her stock response had always been to say she did not know; that she knew her fear was irrational but she could give no reason for it, that it was stupid but real all the same. This time, however, Elizabeth said what she had known all her life.

"Kill me!" She replied. "It will kill me. I have always known it will!"

In the absence of any further information Mr Fellows thought hard about the direction in which Elizabeth should go. The intensity of her fear meant that exposure therapy was out of the question. There were no other chocolate-phobic people that the counsellor was aware of, which meant no group sessions of any kind and there were no medical articles he knew of on Elizabeth's condition.

He eventually reasoned that if Elizabeth's fears could not be countered on a conscious level without causing distress, they might well be countered on an unconscious level. He advised hypnotherapy and made Elizabeth an appointment with a reputable practitioner for the following week.

Dr Carrick Graham was a medical practitioner as well as a hypnotherapist. His usual method of treatment was to gently regress his patient to the point in their life when some personally traumatic event had initiated the fear that eventually became their phobia.

The trigger event could be as simple as a TV programme showing snakes or as distressing as involvement in an accident. Whatever the reason there always was one and the trick was to gently probe the buried memories of the patient and allow them to confront their fears whilst in a relaxed hypnotic state. The good doctor's whole treatment plan was built around this philosophy and his success rate, whilst not perfect, was certainly impressive. He had read thoroughly the notes passed on to him from both Elizabeth's doctor and counsellor and knew roughly what he would search for.

Try as he might Dr Graham could not find a trigger event. He regressed Elizabeth to her very earliest memories and found that the fear was with her even then, as though it was an integral part of her, some component of her genetic make-up. She presented as a fascinating and unique patient.

He probed and teased her memories in the hopes of finding some connection between actions and perception but to no avail. He was at a loss to find some way of helping his patient and was about to tell her so when Elizabeth provided the answer to her own problem.

"It would be wonderful," she said one day as she was about to leave his office, "if there was a world without, *you know what*, a world in which I could be as normal as everyone else, a *thingy*-free world just for me."

That was the answer. A chocolate-free world in which Elizabeth French could function as well as the next person, no fears, no restricted lifestyle, just normality for once in her besieged life. And he could give her that world!

Their next session was to prove the turning point in Elizabeth's life. Once he had relaxed her and induced in her a hypnotic state he told her quite simply that she could not see chocolate. He planted in her mind the mechanism whereby she would block out chocolate, its wrappings, its scent, the very word. She would, he told her, become unaware of its existence; a mental 'cut and delete' in order to protect her sanity.

Before bringing Elizabeth out of her hypnotic state Dr Graham unwrapped a bar of chocolate and placed it in plain view on his desk. He then returned Elizabeth to the here-and-now and began a general conversation with her. She did not see the chocolate. Even when he picked it up and moved it about the desk she carried on talking as though it did not exist. He introduced one or two words and phrases into the conversation; chocolate, Mars, flake, Easter egg, and though a puzzled look crossed her face now and then she seemed not to recognise the words. She picked up where she thought it made sense to and carried on talking.

And so began a new era in the life of Elizabeth French, it was as though her past life had been nothing but an unpleasant dream. She went shopping for the first time in years. Went to the supermarket, walked down the aisle stuffed with sweets and chocolate and never turned a hair.

She drank coffee at the same table as a fat child who crammed a whole chocolate-covered donut into his mouth and never saw it. She bought a beautiful chocolate brown blouse and pale mocha slacks without feeling the slightest bit sick. She went dancing, met a man, invited him back to her apartment and had beautiful, all consuming sex for the first time in years and when he expressed the desire to dip her in chocolate and lick her clean she moaned and sighed and never heard a word of it.

Her new life was complete and she enjoyed every wonderful, joyous, short moment of it.

It was only two weeks after her 'cure' that she crossed the road to meet a friend for coffee. She never saw the vehicle as it bore down on her, though witnesses later said that she was looking straight at it. Her mind was unaware of its presence as it ploughed into her and tossed her into the autumn air as though she was a rag doll.

She never saw the words emblazoned on the cab of the truck as it ended her life.

She never saw *Cadbury's Removals*. Never saw it at all.

Tom Bryan

Road Man

I've kissed ditches, man,
used drain pipes for pillows,
snored under dying stars.
Counted Orion down and out
in the cat-slippered sunrise.

And where the road met the moon,
I pissed human steam on frozen stone,
kept moving to starve the cold,
colliding with the sun
as it called forth serpents
to share my journey.

Kitchen Rat

He limped like a crippled blackbird,
I put a trap down, he stole the bait.
Put down sweet poison,
he ate.

Today I must howk
his remains (or not) out to daylight
with a fire poker.

I'll fear a dead rat
more than a living one.
Maybe because of the limp,
the Sunday rain, or my own
need for dark shadows.

My Mantelpiece

Clown juggles for a driftwood lion,
children smile to a walnut owl.
An Ojibway card thanks me: "Megweetch."
Niece no longer child
grins into her future.

A half century ago
I hold my brother's hand,
our photo propped up by a fossil.

Tom Bryan

Higher above, under a pewter owl,
skeletal jaws (small for a shark)
but big enough to swallow
our memories whole.

Rush Hour
In Front of the Museum of the American Indian (New York City)

Long legs pound like silken jackhammers,
high heels rattle snare drums home.
A swish of insight into market futures,
over website cocktails.

And I feel fat in my crumpling jeans,
lurking out where bagmen prowl
and Rain Forest refugees
peddle wooden flutes.

Eyes deeper than all despair
mumble me for the time
and don't even wait for an answer.

January Night, Selkirk

Cat breath fogs
my window pane, purrs
for any warming door.

Stars rivet chimney pots.
Frosty gloves
smoor streetlights.

Gospel skites
down cobblestones.
Wind belts blues,
my gas fire moans.

Next door,
junkshop spade and picks
crave navvy-sweated yesterdays

and rat piss calendars
remember long-dead women
with lips like slit wrists.

Maurice J. Ryan
Mountain Interlude

Mrs Ofelenia, the wife of the owner of the Negros Occidental Sugar Mill, one of the biggest in the Philippines, hurried down the steps of her villa to meet us. "How kind of you to come to my birthday party," she said warmly, smiling at me and my husband, Arturo, a newly appointed junior manager. "I'm always pleased to meet new staff. What a lovely family you have." She leaned forward and beamed at our three young girls. They were dressed immaculately in expensive pineapple fibre dresses with flounced sleeves in the Filipino Spanish style.

My husband smiled politely at his employer's wife. "It's nice to be able to meet you and your husband socially, ma'am."

At the mention of her husband, the woman's face fell. "I'm sorry, but Ramon isn't back yet. He was called to an urgent meeting with the governor two hours ago. I'm afraid we'll have to start without him. Come and meet the other guests."

She led us to a tiled patio which looked out on to the garden. It was that magical half hour before dusk in the Philippines when everything is bathed in mysterious shadows and colors are etched boldly in rich hues. The guests were being entertained by a troupe of traditional Filipino dancers. They were performing a native Igorot dance from Bontoc Province in Northern Luzon, in which they spread their arms and flapped them slowly up and down like the wings of mountain birds. When the dancing finished, Mrs Ofelenia led the guests into the dining room where the tables were laden wth a variety of Filipino-Spanish delicacies such as Pastel de Lengua, beef-tongue pie, and Pastillas de Leche, a carabao-milk and sugar confection.

The maids were already pouring the coffee in the sala, when Mr Ofelenia suddenly burst into the room, his face as white as a sheet. "The entire Philippine sugar industry has collapsed," he shouted hysterically.

"Calm down, dear," his wife said gently. "Sit down and try to tell us what has happened."

Everyone stared at them both, horrorstruck. We were all only too aware that throughout 1984, the previous year, President Marcos and his financial adviser, Roberta Benedicto, had been buying up sugar from the Negros plantation owners at prices way below its market value. They had then stored it in warehouses all over the island, and waited for the world price to peak so they could resell it and make a huge profit for themselves.

Mr Ofelenia began to speak again, his eyes burning with anger. "Ferdinand Marcos and those other greedy bastards in Manila have miscalculated," he shouted. "The price of sugar on the world market has crashed instead of going up. Our sugar is now unsaleable. We're all out of a job."

The party broke up in disarray. The following day, my husband was laid off work without any severance pay, and we were given five days to vacate our company-owned apartment. "What on earth are we going to do, Arturo?" I said tearfully, when he broke the news to me. "We've no savings to fall back on and we've three young kids to provide for."

My husband shrugged. "If we don't want to starve, our only chance is to move to Manila," he said firmly. "At least there's a chance of getting employment there."

"But where are we going to stay? You know as well as I do that the cost of renting anywhere in Manila is prohibitive, especially if you don't have money in the bank."

Arturo stared at me, apprehension showing in his eyes. "We'll just have to become squatters for a while like thousands of others from the provinces."

"Squatters?" I said, aghast. "You mean you expect me and the children to scrape along in some rat-infested shanty town? You must be crazy."

"No I'm not. Other people do it. I've done my homework on this. Our best bet is to settle in Smokey Mountain near the port in Tondo. There are lots of jobs going in the docks. I'd be bound to find something."

A week later, we sailed from Negros to Manila and arrived at Tondo with our three children and all our belongings crowded into the back of a jeepney. "There's Smokey Mountain," my husband suddenly shouted, as if he was showing me a tourist attraction.

In the distance, to the right, was a grey escarpment of incinerating garbage about three hundred feet high stretching as far as the eye could see. It rose gradually in tiers to a tiny plateau which served as a summit. Squatter huts were clustered on the slopes like blow-flies on a festering wound.

"How can you expect me to live here?" I screamed at Arturo, pointing to the tendrils of smoke from burning rubbish which were curling upwards into the polluted air. "It's like a scene from hell. I don't want to stay here."

My husband looked at me helplessly. "Be reasonable, Angie. They've promised us a makeshift house on the other side, away from the smoke. At least give it a chance. We've no other choice."

"All right," I said, looking at our sweating children, who were already beginning to cough because of the acrid fumes blowing down from the Mountain. "I'll give it two weeks. That's all I can promise."

The first week was a nightmare. At night, huge rats ran across the floor of our makeshift shanty which was made of scraps of corrugated iron and discarded cardboard packing cases. Arturo's previous hopes of getting a job as a driver at the docks proved illusory. The syndicate which controlled the hiring of drivers insisted on a two thousand pesos placement fee which we could not afford. The only work he could get was part-time scavenging for scrap materials on the garbage dump for a few pesos a day.

One morning, at the start of the second week, as I was carrying water from a standpipe to our hut at the top of the escarpment, a man came up to me. He was in his mid-thirties with thick black hair slickly coiffured above his weasel face. It was his clothes however which really stood out. He was wearing immaculate Levi jeans and a flashy silk shirt which looked completely out of place.

"Hi, kummadre," he drawled. "My name's Rudi Gonzalez. I'm recruiting waitresses for a restaurant in Ermita, the tourist belt in town. The pay's three hundred pesos a week, plus tips. Interested?"

I put my water container down on the ground and faced him. "Yes, but I'll need to talk to my husband first."

Arturo was standing outside our shanty, staring vacantly into space, when we arrived. He didn't need much persuading. "I'll take care of the kids while you're at work," he promised.

A taxi dropped me outside the El Dorado Restaurant in Ermita that evening. I was wearing my best dress, sprinkled with perfume to drown the pervasive stench of smoke that polluted everything on Smokey Mountain.

As I entered the brightly lit building, I soon realised that it was a sizeable casino with its own restaurant adjacent to the gaming section. The place was already full of tourists. Several waitresses in green and yellow uniforms were hurrying back and forth around the crowded tables. In the centre was a circular disco where some couples were dancing. I was introduced to the headwaiter, who gave me a green dress, briefly explained my duties and then put me to work right away.

One evening, about a week after I had begun working there, Arturo took me on one side just as I was leaving for work. I could tell he had something on his mind.

"Angie" he said hesitantly, "The foreman down at the port told me he could give me a job as a driver tomorrow if I gave him fifteen hundred pesos. Round here, bribing people is the only way to get places. So d'you think you could ask the manager for an advance on your salary. It would mean an awful lot to me."

"Okay", I said, "I'll ask the boss but I can't promise anything."

Later that evening, after most of the meals had been served, I went along to see Mr Mendoza, the owner of the casino, who lived on his own in a penthouse above the restaurant. I had been warned by the other waitresses to be careful with him. He had a reputation of seducing pretty female employees and then summarily sacking them when they later became pregnant. Moreover, during the previous few days, I had noticed him eyeing me.

Just as I was about to knock on his door, it flew open, and one of the dancers from the floor show came out. She was buttoning up her dress and her hair was in disarray. The casino owner was standing in the doorway behind her. He was wearing an expensive silk dressing gown and was holding a white poodle in his arms. As soon as he saw me, his eyes lit up.

"Hello, gorgeous," he said, brushing back a wisp of grey hair from his balding forehead, "What can I do for you?" He remained in the doorway, holding his protuding stomach. I began to tell him about my problem but felt uneasy since his roving eyes were scanning my body like an X-ray machine. He reminded me of a fat anaconda that was eyeing its next meal.

"An advance on your salary?" he said with a smirk, showing his tobacco-stained teeth. "You must be joking. I don't give favours like that for nothing, at least not to pretty women like you. You can't expect that sort of money on a plate. I'afraid you'll have to give me a bit of fun first. Understand?"

"What sort of fun exactly?" I stammered, realising the full enormity of the dilemma he was facing me with.

Still holding the poodle, he walked over to the door of his adjacent bedroom and pointed to the king-sized bed. At each corner, were leather straps, and on the bedtable was a horse whip. "Strap me to the bed and whip me until I beg you to stop," he said, "and I'll give you one thousand pesos in cash outright."

I simply stared at him, overcome with revulsion. "Is that all?" I said hesitantly.

"Yes, that's all. You can go after that, and get on with your work downstairs."

What he was asking was against my deepest moral convictions. For an instant I just looked at him, wondering to do. Then I thought of my children slowly suffocating to death amid the pollution of Smokey Mountain and the way my husband was unable to get a steady job as a driver. "Okay, I'll do it," I said, "but nothing else, you understand, and I want cash in advance, now."

The man's reptile face lit up with anticipation. Reaching in his pocket he pulled out his wallet and handed me two crisp five hundred pesos bills. Then he pointed to the straps. "Fasten them tightly round both my hands and feet so that I can't move an inch. Then whip me as hard as you can. I've been a naughty boy, so you'll need to give me a really good hiding."

Just as he was unfastening the belt of his dressing gown, the door was suddenly flung open and three tough-looking men wearing denims and T-shirts burst into the room. As I stood there, frozen with fear, they took out a handgun each and walked casually up to the owner of the casino. The leader stood in front of him.

"Chico Mendoza?"

The man nodded.

"We're cadres of a Sparrow Unit of the revolutionary New People's Army of the Philippines. You're an enemy of the people. Do you have anything to say before we pass sentence?"

Mendoza stared at him defiantly. "It's a free country. I've done nothing wrong. Go to hell."

"Nothing wrong eh? You spend most of your time debasing and exploiting Filipinos working for you like this poor lady here and yet you insist you're innocent?"

Suddenly, he looked at me. "Get out of here and take that with you," he said, pointing to the man's wallet lying on the bedside table. "He won't be needing it any more."

Just as I reached the end of the corridor, I heard the shots. As I hurried down the stairs, I looked inside the wallet. It was stuffed with hundred dollar bills. My interlude on Smokey Mountain was over.

Mike Marqusee

Aesthetic

Spare me the wallet-thumpers and mickey-takers,
spare me the shyness of men in suits,
spare me the tears of movers and shakers,
spare me the hollow sound of flutes.

Give me something boisterous, something bohemian
something potable – cool and long and lush –
give me the downside, give me comedians,
give me that methedrine rush.

Make it sarcastic, make it ebullient,
make it tremble in the heat,
make it breathe with giant lungs,
make it nullify defeats.

Sculpt the lover's cheeks and hollows,
print the tabloid tale of grief,
strike it out in nervous colours,
strike it out in bold relief.

Make it extreme cause the world is extreme,
but make it gentle and evanescent,
cut and paste cartoons and dreams,
sample the fibrous, delirious, edible present.

The Cat in the Hat

My head was buried in the Leominster Herald,
life in the provinces had swallowed me up,
the Corn Square was being pedestrianised,
drug dealers and small floods were pestering
long-time residents, and the Classic Car Society
had cancelled its monthly meeting when

suddenly there was incense of charred mutton, the brisk
taste of buttermilk on my breath and I saw
a Pukhtoon hat pulled down
over the ears of a white man with a moustache,
a beaky nose and an itinerant's strut
– elbows flaring, eyes swivelling, knees at the ready –
that made me think in his time he had hacked his way
through the multitudinous cities of the south.

Mike Marqusee

He was whispering to a young woman
in black leggings and a tired jumper
whose little laughs left puffs of vapour.
I liked the way he wore that hat.
The round flat crown with the smooth nap
sloped cunningly so that the roll
perched over the eyebrows
possibly hiding hair loss or who knows
some mildly offensive tattoo.

Had he haggled for that hat
in a smugglers' camp round a paraffin stove?
Did he pay too much on a package tour?
Did he salute when he heard the name Khan Abdul Gaffar Khan?

I knew that hat, had seen it
on politicians, peasants, chess players
across the North West Frontier Province,
and it made me smile
as I remembered Zain-ud-din Khilji,
a devout Sunni who ran a family planning clinic in Quetta.

I wanted to stop, say out loud
how much I dug the lid,
but the man with the Pukhtoon hat
was sticking his grey tongue in his companion's ear
and the forecast in the Herald was for more of the same.

Old Mose Knows
(Monument Valley, 1994)

He's wandered among the red pinnacles
since the early fifties, eaten dirt, dressed
as a woman, laughed off heat and hunger.

Doffing his trademark sombrero
he makes a start, gets stuck for words
falls back on a catchphrase, dimly recalled.

"Thank'ye kindly, Ethan, thank'ye kindly . . ."
His master has passed on.
John Ford in black sunglasses

measuring the daylight
swirling down the canyons, mixing
patience with impatience, made this void

poignant, a rendezvous of peoples,
a test
of allegiance.

Old Mose was left behind.
His skull is brown.
He's giddy with loneliness.

He will be my guide
through this civilisation of stone.
He will thread the teetering steeples

and scamper the battlements
where the towers are blind,
where the giants whisper and play.

Old Mose knows.
I have tracked him to his lair.
"Thank'ye kindly, Ethan, thank'ye kindly."

I study my shadow.
It looms like a statue.
It has Big Shoulders like John Wayne.

Apologia with muttered aside

I'm here to tell you that the lift
will continue not to work, the damp
will spread incrementally and the waiting list
for transfers is longer than the M1.

I'm here to tell you that your tips
will be deemed taxable income
and deducted from your wages.

I'm here to tell you that your Housing Benefit
will be withheld, your dinner party
boycotted, and your funeral banned.

Mike Marqusee

I'm here to tell you that a white
fungus will grow between your toes but
your allotment will be barren.

I'm here to tell you that your friend who laughs
aloud while he cooks exotic meals will die
slowly of a sickness ultimately stripping him
of his sense of humour and shrivelling
his taste buds.

(You don't like it? It's my job,
scumbag, you think I give
a fuck what you say?
What makes you better than me?
In your dreams, Holy Joe!)

I'm here to tell you that your enemies
have been appointed poll watchers,
the ballot is rigged but the elections
will be declared free and fair.

Song of the Besieged

Drink yourself silly tonight, the news is bad:
riots have broken out among the rich and famous,
they're heading our way in a raucous rabble,
they're heading our way seeking revenge.

Let's have a pint and a chaser each,
count our offences and prepare to amend
whatever it is that's maddened the pack,
whatever it is makes them slaver and pant.

It's dark outside but in here there's beer,
fags in the machine and nothing to lose,
the only complaint the price of a double,
the only sound the hubbub that soothes.

So what if somewhere in this city tonight
troubled millionaires go red in the face,
form posses in search of a good night's sleep,
form victim support groups and beg for relief?

Have you ever noticed how sensitive they are,
the famously famous, to wisecracks and quips,
how quick to react to a fall in the pound,
how adept at assessing the stranger's kiss?

Poor darlings! Having to remember
the innumerable names of unfamiliar friends,
having to remember to speak for us all
yet never speak ill of the lame or the dead.

So the news is bad, they're lonely and mean,
the rich and famous from *Hello* magazine.
Our betters are demented but after one more short
we forgive their excesses and turn to the sport.

Morag Hadley

Immortelle

The first time Grace saw the angel he was playing a golden horn and standing on top of a carved sarcophagus. Grace had noticed one or two of them dotted about the cemetery, but she'd never seen a black angel before. His skin glowed, like honey melting on a silver spoon, and thick, black eyelashes fluttered on cheekbones as smooth as whalebone as he executed a particularly high note on his horn. He was wearing loose black trousers and a white shirt with billowing sleeves.

"You seen my husband?" Grace shouted. "Hey, you. You up there, you seen my hubby?" The angel didn't reply. He raised his golden horn skywards and played, "*Falling in love with you.*" Grace hummed one or two bars; she'd forgotten the words. She might have tried a few dance steps as well but her feet hurt.

The angel turned to her and said, "Cat got your tongue?" Not sharply, she thought. The words came out all gentle, slow and warm, unfurling themselves from his pink tongue, as if they came from somewhere deep inside him or, from very far away.

"He should be here somewhere. I've been looking ever such a long time."

"Probably hiding," the angel said. "Should be lots of places to hide here, I should think." Grace didn't like to say that if an angel didn't know all the hiding places in Larchwood Grange cemetery then who would, and that it was a daft thing to say. She was tired. The gatekeeper had given her more cheek than usual. One of these days she'd report him. Maybe a word with the black angel would help. Perhaps he could fix things.

"Here, help me up," Grace panted. "Might see him from up there beside you." She thrust her shopping bag at the angel who swooped up both the bag and Grace so fast that she was standing on the tombstone before she knew how she'd got there. The marble, which needed a good cleaning, she noted, cooled her feet a treat.

"You can see the whole world from here," he said.

"Betcha can't." What a daft thing for an angel to say, she thought. Why would an angel have to get up on top of a tombstone to see the whole world? He blew a few toots on his golden horn that sounded to Grace a bit like, "*I'm Sitting on Top of the World.*"

"Here, pass my bag." Grace was about to say, "there's a good boy" but managed to stop herself in time, and asked his name instead.

"Bilbo," he said. Now what sort of a name was that for an angel? Something like Benedict or Benjamin would be appropriate – Barrabus at a pinch.

"Hey, what's in this, lady?" Bilbo asked, setting down her shopping bag, "How d'you manage to carry it?" Grace had never been called lady by anyone, but it felt extra special coming from an angel. To think of all the times she'd been here and never seen him.

"Picnic. I always bring a picnic for us. My husband likes a bit of ham and pickle." Her eyes swept the skyline. The angel was right. There was a view. Not the whole world, but she could see the river winding its way under Hammersmith bridge, towards the sea. "Here. Help me up, Bilbo."

"But you've just sat down, lady." There it was again. Lady. Later, back in the flat, she'd practise the way the angel said it so that she could tell the butcher that's what she'd like to be called instead of Missus. Bilbo helped her up, one firm hand on her elbow, the other grasping her hand. Grace couldn't help noticing that his fingers were long and tapered like wings, except that they were black. Funny, she'd never thought of angels having black wings.

"To see the sea. I might see the sea if I stand up," she told him.

"Oh, I don't think so. Sea's a long way . . ."

". . . I might. I might just see it. We like the sea, my hubby and I. Nice picnics at the seaside." Now, why did the angel say that? Seeing the sea should be an easy thing for an angel to arrange. Grace's eyes were beginning to get blurry, the way they always did when she was upset. "Date sandwiches at the seaside. Date and sand sandwiches Reg used to call them."

"Well, why not?" the black angel said, "why shouldn't a lady see the sea?" And with a great flourish of his golden horn he began to play, *"Oh, I do like to be beside the seaside."* As he played, his eyes sparkled, but Grace didn't notice as hers gently closed. The traffic noise faded; instead, she heard the tumble and drag of pebbles on the beach, and Reg's voice, way off key, trying hard not to laugh, finishing off, ". . . *beside the sea-e-e.*"

✶✶

"'Cept – we can't see it. Gracie, can we?" They huddled together in a wooden shelter on the promenade. Reg's arm was tight around her shoulder, the other one round her waist, tucked into her winter coat. Her hands were clamped between his knees to keep them warm, and his uniform, as hairy as gooseberries, tickled. She didn't mind the wind and rain. They were together. That was all that mattered. "Here, cuddle in, Gracie. Got any of them sandwiches left?" His hand moved easily from her waist and encircled her breast. She felt his ragged nails dragging at the soft, cobwebby wool of her new jumper, but that didn't matter either. It felt just right on her, firm and, and . . . well, just right.

"Pilchards. They're pilchards," she said.

"Well, never mind, eh Gracie. We're out of the wind here. Perishing. Some bloody embarkation leave. A ruddy gale."

"Such a shame, Reg. Should've been different. I did so want it to be special."

"But it is, my Gracie. What about last night in the Sea Spray guest

house? Forgotten already, have you? If that wasn't pretty special . . ." Grace was glad it was dark and Reg couldn't see the hot flush she felt on her cheeks.

Last night, when Reg was rocking and touching her, and kissing every bit of her, she'd forgotten all about the lies she'd told Mum. When he made love to her she'd forgotten how cold it was, and that the landlady's sheets were damp. She forgot everything except that Reg loved her. Being loved by Reg was the best thing that had ever happened to Gracie; better than the night they'd met at the Hammersmith Palais. "You're my shimmering butterfly" he'd whispered in her ear as they danced under the spinning silver globe. And, last night, he'd made her feel as if she was hovering on the edge of something really wonderful.

"Oh Reg, I wish, I wish you didn't have to."

"C'mon, duck, we said we wouldn't mention that. We came to see the sea and there it is." He pointed with his sandwich. "Go on. Look." Grace couldn't see a thing, just mist and rain. She didn't know what she'd do with Reg gone.

"Can't see a thing," she sniffled. "You're having me on."

"I promised you the sea. Now, close your eyes like a good girl and you'll see it."

Hidden in the shelter, in the mist, with her eyes closed, waiting to see the sea, gently, ever so gently. Reg undid the rest of her coat buttons then opened his greatcoat, and gathered her so close into him she could barely breathe. Their bodies rose and fell in time with the soughing wind and the sound of pebbles rumbling, like sweets in a jar. Rising and falling, with Reg. By the sea.

**

"Can you see it? Is it sparkling and blue?" For a moment the angel's whispering voice sounded just like Reg.

"No. No . . . but I can imagine it, can't I?" Feeling cold, Grace pulled the edges of her blue coat together. "I can imagine it, so I'll see it in my what's-it. My . . ."

"Mind's eye," a little puff of breath from the angel said.

"That's it. My mind's eye." Grace looked sideways at the angel. He was a clever angel, she'd say that for him.

Grace was surprised that angel Bilbo had eaten three sandwiches. Not that she grudged him – she was just surprised, him being an angel and all.

"Your husband's missing out a bit here. Grace. Nice sandwiches these."

"He won't mind. Told you, didn't I? He's all right, is my hubby." The marble slab had warmed up in the sun. Maybe that's why the angel came. She'd read that ice formed on the wings of 'planes, so perhaps angels had the same problem.

"The stone's nice and warm. That why you come here?"

"No, it reminds me of my Grandmother."

"She's not under her, is she? We're never sitting on top of your Gran havin' a picnic?" Grace stood up, ready to jump down, when the angel reassured her that the twisted columns beneath them looked just like his Gran's dining table's legs, and that they were sitting on top of someone called Sir Claudius Permenter. What a mouthful! Trust toffs to have Claudius for a name, not Claude like ordinary folks. The angel must have read her thoughts. He said,

"What's your husband's name then, Grace?"

"Where is he? That's what I'd like to know. Where is he all this time? Not right of him to go off like that. Not right at all. Can't see him anywhere. You seen him?" She turned to Bilbo. "You seen my husband?" She stood up. "You can almost see the sea from here." She sang, her voice crackling, "*Oh, I do like to be beside the seaside. Oh I do like to be beside . . .*" Gently, Bilbo helped her sit down again. Grace watched, her heart going all pit-a-pat, as the angel put his golden horn to his dark, peony coloured lips and began to play, "*Hush little Baby.*" When he'd finished playing he said,

"C'mon, Lady Grace, we'll look together. He'll be here somewhere."

"Reginald."

"What's that, Grace?"

"His name. Only I call him Reg. He's more of a Reg."

"Not a Claudius, then, Grace?" Bilbo said, and Grace laughed with him. He was a clever angel. Bilbo lifted her down. Ever so gently, like she was something precious. Little crystals – no, they must be diamonds – sparkled around the edges of his thick, curly hair. Grace wanted to reach out and touch them, but didn't. Wasn't proper. They set off across the grass, Bilbo playing a Sousa march to help them along. It made her feel ever so proud to have such a good-looking angel by her side.

"Look, that might be him," Bilbo cried. "That man on the bench. I'll go and see." And he bounded off, skimming across the grass in his white boots which, Grace couldn't help noticing, had useful blue wings down each side. How clever. His white shirt billowed behind him, like a sail. If she was lucky, Grace thought, as she trotted along behind, she might catch a peep of his glossy, black wings. She started to puff a bit and wished that the angel would slow down. It was all very well for him, with winged feet and all. The oompah-pahs, from the angel's golden horn, instead of becoming fainter, as he flew on ahead, got louder and louder – so loud that they made Grace's head ache. She felt herself coming over all giddy.

**

"*The full name, Miss,*" the man behind the high, polished counter repeated. "*We require full name, rank and serial number.*" His voice hissed as he emphasised "*Miss.*"

Gracie told him again, trying to shut out the rousing music that came from the military band, and cheers from the crowd, three streets away, that Reg's name was Reginald Stanley Franklin, and that he was a mechanic in the Royal Engineers. Didn't seem right, all these celebrations and Reg not back. "When did you last hear from him?" Gracie couldn't tell the man that she hadn't heard a dicky bird – not since he'd loved her and turned her into a glittery butterfly, in the middle of winter, by the sea. "What a little fool," he would say. Like Mum, he would say, "what a little fool."

**

She was cross with angel Bilbo for even thinking that the man on the bench could possibly have been Reg. Reg would never wear a cap. Snappy dresser was Reg. Nothing but the best for you and me, Gracie. Nothing but the best, he would say. She'd caught her breath, and was just about to give the angel a telling off when she caught sight of Reg.

"Look, Bilbo! Over there. Standing by that grave. Among the flowers. Him in the hat. That'll be Reg. In 'is hat." Grace grabbed the angel's cool hand and flew across the grass as if she'd never had a day's rheumatism in her life.

It wasn't Reg, after all, but they'd joined the mourners anyway, who didn't seem to mind. Would add a bit of class. Grace thought, having an angel at a funeral. Angel Bilbo hadn't minded that it was a bit of a busman's holiday for him. Lovely voice too. Grace couldn't help thinking that it was a great pity that Bilbo was an angel. Bit of a waste, really.

"Lovely hymn that." Grace settled herself down on top of their tombstone. "My favourite, *'Abide with Me.'* Says such a lot, that hymn."

"It certainly does, Lady Grace." Bilbo's mouth was full of Grace's home-made gingerbread; his voice was thick, like plush velvet, like the treacle in the gingerbread. Lady Grace! Oh my. Wait 'til Reg hears.

"*Fight the Good Fight,*" Grace announced, suddenly.

"Ye-es. That too." He sounded doubtful. Grace thought Bilbo would've known all about hymns.

"Reg's favourite. That's what he'd want. Here, have another cuppa."

"When's that, Grace?"

"For 'is send-off, of course. You know," she said, nodding back to where the mourners were still gathered. "Out with a bang. That's what Reg says. Out with a bang."

**

She sat in the same shelter and watched the fireworks at the end of the pier. Gracie was glad it was dark and she couldn't see the sea. It's sparkling would've made her eyes ache. She already had a headache from all the booms, crackles and bangs of the celebration fireworks. She looked and looked for Reg in the streams of laughing people strolling along the promenade. She listened for his firm tread among the clattering high heels and brown brogues. She watched out for his brown trilby. There were black and grey hats by the dozen passing by their shelter, sitting high on ugly heads, full of laughing teeth, too happy, far too happy at being here, by the sea. Counting them in the dark made her head ache so.

**

"Don't cry. Grace. We'll hand in the hat at the gate." For a moment. Grace thought Bilbo meant '*the pearly gates*,' because she felt ever so queer, all light headed, with stars exploding somewhere behind her eyes, as if she'd forgotten to take her pills. They were sitting on top of Sir Claudius: a rather battered looking silk top hat lay between them. Grace's cheeks were sopping wet with tears, and the angel was mopping them up with his shirt sleeves, and patting her on the back at the same time.

"He gets that all the time. I've seen it happen all the time here. I've seen lots of old ladies knock hats off undertakers." Bilbo smiled. If she'd had a son, Grace decided, she'd have wanted him to be just like Bilbo.

"Too big for Reg. Far too big. Anyhow, he'd never wear black. Never." Grace watched an empty hearse go through the main gate, vaguely remembering a lot of shouting and arm waving, by people dressed in black. Good riddance, she thought.

"Here. Help me up."

"You sure? Be dark soon, Lady Grace. I'll need to be leaving soon."

"I want to look at the stars before I go. Reg knows all about them. Says that he's got as many kisses for me as there are stars. I want to stand up and see the stars – and remember."

"Remember what, Grace?" Bilbo said, his voice an angel's whisper.

"Not quite dark enough for stars yet." But Grace knew better. Bilbo was the best angel she could ever hope to meet, but he didn't know everything.

"I want to stand up here and see the stars. I saw the sea, and I'll see the stars too. I know I will." She stood very still. The angel's fluttering sleeves made little flapping noises, like bunting strung from a flagpole. His lips were pursed, as pretty as a baby's, ready to play, and the tune that he played for his Lady Grace was, sweet and haunting, and was called "*Starry, Starry Night*," and though Grace didn't know this she might have guessed.

"When I see the stars I'll remember everything . . . everything I want to remember," and Grace gazed towards the heavens and waited.

When she spoke again, her voice was that of a young woman. Bilbo's notes strung themselves across the silver-blue wings of the evening sky, catching her words as she spoke.

"I can see them. The stars. One, by one, they're coming out. I can see them ever so clearly. Look! There. And there. Out they come, sparkly bright. One, by one, by one. They're all there. Millions of them, bursting into my mind's eye. I can see everything. I can remember everything! And here's Reg, bless him. Knew I'd see him. Knew I'd remember. Knew I'd see everything in my, in my . . ."

"Mind's eye. Grace. Your mind's eye," Bilbo whispered.

Art Work

The artwork ends up here en route to the car boot sale;

1
Sun punished landscapes
that take up too much space
like the woman who mumbles
on the rush hour bus does.

2
Adolescent skies
that fade into the institutional blue
painted round the dining room
to make the food, taste.

3
In the kitchen above the bread bin
between a health and hygiene certificate
and a Times Roman note that reads:
"Please turn kettle off at wall"
a surreal fruit bowl sulks like an oily teenager,

another staff masterpiece from a last chance night class
unframed, unsigned.

Susan

She sits, still as an exam,

blue bottle painted nails, quiet hair.
She says her name is Susan and,
I believe her.

She asks for mine but I don't answer,

want to see if silence scares her,
she sits, still enough to touch.

Bernadette Cremin

For now she is convenient, somewhere to park questions
feel uneasy with, nearly laugh.

For now, she is enough of me to like
some of someone else,
and something I don't need to know.

Thin Curtain

I went to bed early last night
with the cello-tape-spine paperback
that I underline in green,
scribble in the margins
as if coaxing something out.

Our unmade bed room smelt of excuses
and kicked off shoes,
so I lit a stick of sandalwood:
watched its slender smoke
trace the mix-n-match furniture
that we've cluttered with mug rings,
and top-lost cosmetic bottles,
and the contents of your emptied pocket;
sixteen pence in loose change, wallet, keys
and today's till receipt from Sainsburys
for the usual: egg roll, cherry coke, King size Twix.

I went to bed early last night
leaving you to grope the evening
for stimulating company on your own
afforded by late night b rate pornography
and blended whiskey.

You trip-tip-toed in late
I feigned sleep to avoid another faked headache
and watched you undress in the voyeuristic streetlight
that sneaks in through the thin curtain
that can't hide either side anymore.

Bernadette Cremin

Quarry Tiles

He's spilt her on the kitchen floor.

She lies, curled toward the sun
watching the warm leak from her temple
crawl toward the door
like a fat worm.

He goes upstairs, changes his shirt,
leaving her to count the 98 stripes in the curtain again,
the hem still needs mending,
she'll get some red cotton, tomorrow.

She hears the cough,
phlegm-spit-in-the-toilet-flush,
knows he'll be back in 27 steps
to smoke a Marlboro to the filter,
sink another Tenants Extra
then go out, anywhere.

When he leaves she'll drink tea
with the dirty breakfast things

and then mop up the mess
before the kids get in from school.

High Ceiling

The ceiling

is farther away, when you can't walk to the door.

Owen Dwyer

Greed

The road of excess leads to the palace of wisdom
William Blake

"Don't you think that's a bit self indulgent? I mean, you're killing yourself, ruining your life for a momentary pleasure."

"Self-indulgent? Don't talk to me about self-indulgence," she rasped leaving me disliking her even more. I was riddling my drunk brain for a response when she continued: "You come in here drunk, carrying a curry and a kebab and chips, and six cans of cider."

The kebab was for Joe; he had insisted I buy it as we left the pub. This despite him going back to Rosie's flat. Some English Rosie, who lived at the end of the yellow brick road that stretched from Dublin to London, who had sex in her flat whenever she felt like it. The curry was for me, the *ruby murray*, bought because I had never tasted Indian food and because the rhyming slang sounded delicious. I was on a week's holidays from the tedium of Dublin and my father's disapproval, if I liked what I saw I was going to stay and look for work. I was on the crest of new experience and could not wait to taste the exotic gunge as I heaved open the broken door of the squat. She was sitting calmly in the dark, not even smoking, two dark eyes staring condescendingly from a colourless face, at me and nothing, concurrently. The crack of light from the door I had left ajar lit her dully.

"Look love," I said. "There's a difference. Getting drunk and eating take-aways is one thing, locking yourself up all day and injecting heroin into your veins is something completely different."

"Is it?" She snapped. "What's the difference?"

"One kills you. The other just gives you a headache and diarrhoea."

"Oh please. Any idiot knows that ten times more people die as a result of alcohol poisoning than heroin abuse. Not to mention the wife beating, car accidents, hooliganism and violence outside clubs and bars. Over eighty per cent of violent crime is attributed to alcohol abuse. You're just off the fucking boat, what would you know? They don't tell you anything in Ireland."

"That's a load of crap."

"Why?"

"No. I mean. Just look at you and your boyfriend. You never go anywhere, you never do anything."

"What's there to do? Where's there to go?"

I snapped the ring on a can of cider, opening it at my second attempt. "Well you could do a day's work, pay your own way."

"Nobody works over here. You and your friends, the Irish drunks. You come over here collecting the dole in different places, screwing the government. And when you do do a day's work, you never pay tax."

"Jesus, it's only the English government. It's not like we owe Thatcher anything."

She settled back into the beanbag, lit a cigarette and blew the plume up to heaven.

"You're really stupid, do you know that?" I resented the revelation. She was too clever for me to challenge head on, I knew that she was looking for a confrontation in her bored midnight; her boyfriend comatose on a mattress upstairs and me the red-faced virgin fresh off the boat.

"You're really stupid," she repeated. "If you think there is any point to work. What did your parents ever get out of work? A lifetime of slaving to pay the mortgage on a semi-detached. Ulcers from worrying where the car repayments were going to come from. Scrimping and saving and the only thing they enjoy is getting drunk or making a fool of themselves doing the old time waltz during the disco at some niece's wedding? Work? You fucking idiot."

"So you're saying heroin is an alternative to that; a whole other life?"

"Does it matter what I'm saying? You wouldn't understand anyway. You're mind's already closed." She scowled and sucked.

"Well then. Why don't you tell me what it's like?"

"What?"

"Taking heroin."

"Jesus. Listen to him."

I gulped cider as she smoked in the silence looking indifferent. There was no other movement in the space between us. Her boyfriend, who I had only glimpsed earlier as a mop-haired slouch, remained motionless upstairs. He could have been dead.

"Death. That's what it's all about." She said finally. "Death."

There was more silence. I drank, then smoked and tried to look like I had some clue.

"You know that every time you inject, it could be your last, but you don't care. It's the pleasure. It's like the best orgasm you've ever had, if you've ever really had one, multiplied by ten, by a hundred, all over your body. It completely consumes you. Nothing else matters or ever did, but the pleasure. And the only thing you know is that you've never experienced pleasure like this before and you never will again. I get more pleasure from one hit than you'll get in a lifetime. That's why we do it. We're not trying to be rebels or change the world we just want to be left alone with the pleasure. It doesn't matter where we are or what happens to us or anyone else. Nothing matters. And it's when you reach that nothing matters part you realise what a waste all the rest is. How futile people are, how ridiculous people like you are, your prejudices, your narrow-minded ignorance, your complete incomprehension of everything. Your whole life will be one long drawn out misery. Oh you'll convince yourself that there are high points. The birth of a sprog, meeting some inane bitch you see as your soul mate. But they'll all let you down in time, and you'll let them down. You'll die years from now at the end of a long miserable life. Mine will be ten times shorter but with ten times the enjoyment. I'll have exhausted the pleasure gland and refused to indulge in the misery. It's all to do with time, you want it, I don't."

"Is that it? It's all about pleasure. As simple as that. You're a glutton for pleasure?"

"I'm not the only one am I? You come over here, you and your like, not because you want a career or even to work, but because you want money. You're guests of the nation, abusing its hospitality because of your greed; for money, for sex, for cheap beer, chips and cigarettes. So that you can go back at Christmas acting the big man with all that sex experience and money to burn in your pockets. It's all about ego-satiation, being able to say to your mates that you got laid or that you had an argument with some junkie bitch in a squat and ripped her to shreds. You're trying to denigrate and dismiss me for no other reason than to satiate your fragile ego. But it doesn't matter. I don't give a shit because nothing matters."

I had to keep talking; I did not want her to see how upset I was. "What about your man upstairs? If nothing matters, what are you doing with him?"

She reached her cigarette hand out and nodded at a can of cider, which I opened and handed to her.

"You wouldn't understand."

"You can't keep dismissing my questions by telling me I'm too stupid to understand the answer."

She laughed, a little indulgently, a little scornfully.

"Were in this together, Jim and me. This was his thing and now it's our thing. It's what we do. There's nothing else to it; nothing else to know. Why should you care?"

"You're right. I don't care. I'm going to bed."

"Already? I was half thinking of fucking you."

I did not find her attractive, she was over weight, pale and dirty. I was twenty-two and drunk. She bit and scratched as we made love and made small annoyed noises in the back of her throat. She resented me for not giving her enough pleasure, for not being heroin. Afterwards she returned to her corner and watched as I guzzled the curry.

Years later I met Joe for a drink in Dublin. It was the mid nineties and he had just returned with the receding emigration wave to the economic boom. I asked him about the girl.

"Eimer? The once and famous junkie. She got her act together big time after she had the sprog. Gave up the drugs, left your man Jim behind in the squat. Then he died, the poor fucker. I had to call the ambulance and we all had to get out of the squat. We were interrgated by the police, had to give blood samples and everything."

"Jesus. But tell us, what happened to this Eimer one?"

"As far as I know she ended up getting a job in social services, working with disadvantaged kids or something. Then I heard somewhere she'd married. The funny thing about her was that she was always full of brains. Full of crap but full of brains. The kid really sorted her out, although how poor oul Jim managed to knock her up is a complete mystery."

"Are you sure it was him that knocked her up?"

"Sure who else could it have been? They didn't leave the squat for months."

"Who do you think?" I answered; laughing as amused revelation changed his expression. Then I shut up and gobbled my pint.

Short Biographies

The Main Judges

Poetry

Subhadassi

Subhadassi is a freelance writer. Over the past five years he has undertaken various commissions and residencies. These have included a poetry film script commission, a residency on Newcastle's underground Metro rail network, another at Washington Wildfowl Reserve and a Poetry Society Poetry Places Residency, a drama script commission and several poetry commissions. His full length collection of poems, *peeled*, published by ARC, is due out in 2004.

Fiction

Denise Robertson

Denise has published eighteen novels and a great many short stories. One of her early novels won the Constable Award for fiction. Another was recently made into a stage musical *Fine Fine Fine* and performed before sell-out audiences.

Peter Lister

As well as working on the Biscuit team, Peter's main job is Police Detective. He lives in a rural Northumbrian market town, with his wife and two small daughters. Peter's main interests outside of books are riding his mountain bike, running and listening to music.

The Winning Writers

Derek Adams is a professional photographer living in Essex. Born in East London in 1957. A member of the Southend Poetry Group and an organiser of the Essex Poetry Festival (http://come.to/the-essex-poetry-festival). Poems in: *BoomerangUK, Clean Sheets (USA), Moonstone, Other Poetry, Poetry Nottingham, Poetry Monthly, Strange Horizons (USA), Tears in the Fence* and *Winedark Sea* (Aust.). When not writing he likes to wander around in cemeteries, collect magic lantern slides and drink red wine (not all at the same time!).

Karin Bachmann, born in 1969, is Swiss. She usually writes for children and so far six of her adventure/crime stories have been published in a series designed to spur children's interest in reading. At twenty-one, she began learning English. Since then she has been writing in both German and English.

Andrew Neil Blewitt was born in Erith. After a career in public administration in Kent and Sussex he took early retirement and moved with his wife, Ruth, to Norfolk. Neil writes mostly humorous verse much of which has been published and broadcast. He also contributes, in prose, to freethought journals.

Biographies

Peter Bromley lives and works in the North East of England. He has had work published in *Route, The Echo Room* and *New Voices: North East* amongst other places. In 2002 he won a Northern Promise Award from New Writing North and he thanks them for this help.

Tom Bryan was born in Canada in 1950 but is long resident in Scotland. He is a widely published poet and fiction writer. He works as Arts Development Officer in Caithness in the Scottish Highlands. He is separated, with a grown son and daughter. He plays a bit of harmonica in a duo called "Wolfwind."

Sean Burn is a writer, artist and performer who has toured, exhibited, and been published internationally. His most recent poetry collection is *voltairechoruses* – a collaboration with photographer Andrew Hardie. Theatre commissions include *in an age of double-glazin* for paines plough. He tours Germany this Autumn with work from his unpublished novel *molotovs happy hour*. He is currently writer-in-residence with Half-moon Theatre, London.

Tania Casselle is a freelance features writer from London. Her fiction has been published in literary magazines and in the book anthology *Harlot Red* (Serpent's Tail.) She has received recognition in the Raymond Carver Short Story Award, the Asham Award, and the Santa Fe Writers Project Literary Awards.

Graham Clifford is a graduate of the UEA MA in creative writing, appeared at the Hay Festival, was highly commended in the New Writer Poetry Collection category, runner up in the Arvon/Telegraph competition, both in 2002. Published in numerous magazines (the *Rialto, Smiths Knoll* and *La Rue Bella*), Graham teaches in a primary school in Newham, London.

Bernadette Cremin writes 'page and stage' poetry. Since 2000 she has won a SEA performance bursary, been awarded a YOTA and commission by The South. Bernadette has represented Brighton in national/BBC digital slam and released a spoken word album with State Art. She has been published by Halfpenny, Pulsar, Pathade, Soundings et al and been commended by Blue Nose and SEWEA. She is studying poetry at Sussex University and lives in Brighton with a nosey neighbour and eclectic CD collection.

Owen Dwyer lives in North Dublin where he is a partner in a pension brokerage. He is an award-winning short story writer. *The Agitator*, his first novel is due to be published by PublishBritannica in early 2004. He is married and has four children.

Josephine M. Fagan completed her MA in Creative Writing at UNN last year. Her short stories have been published in several anthologies. She is currently working on a novel and several scripts for the BBC. Josephine lives in Newcastle and works part-time as a doctor and an undergraduate tutor.

Tracey Fuller was a runner up from the 2002 Biscuit Prize. She is writing a novella, to be published by Biscuit in 2004, which takes a lifeboat crew, a vintage car and a diving show through the Great War. She is finishing her Creative Writing MA at Middlesex University as well as finding time, with her husband, to ride Daisy their tandem around Sussex.

Sylvia Goodman wrote a love story when she was fifteen that was read under desks! Since then she has had articles and poems published in various media, including the *Times Educational Supplement* and *Envoi*. Her main interests being theatre and travel, she prefers to write in these fields, but poems slip through the cracks in writer's block.

Morag Hadley started writing when she retired from the British Council. She finds it a great excuse for day dreaming which has plagued her for most of her life. She has received various awards from the SAW, NAWG, Edinburgh University, Real Writers, and Fish Publishing, for short stories, poetry and drama. Morag now lives in Bristol.

John Halladay has been awarded many poetry prizes as well as being published in magazines and anthologies. His first collection, *Letters From Ravensbruck*, is published by the University of Sheffield. He is presently working on a novel. John is married with two children and lives in the south of England.

Ruth Henderson has lived in North Shields all her life where she finds inspiration for her stories in the history and splendour of the area. She discovered that being a first-prize winner of Biscuit 2001 opened doors, particularly with radio producers and magazine editors and now has an agent making interesting noises over a children's novel.

Doreen Hinchliffe was born in West Yorkshire but now lives in London, where she teaches English as a Foreign Language. Her poems have appeared in a number of small magazines and she has also won or been highly commended in several competitions, including the Poetry Life competition and the Petra Kenney Award. Five of her poems were published in last year's Biscuit anthology.

Gordon Hodgeon lives in Teesside, works part-time in education, part-time in poetry, which now includes Hall Garth Poets, Brotton Writers and editorial board of Mudfog Press. His last collection was *A Cold Spell* (Mudfog 1996). Other poems recently published in *Penniless Press*, *Red Sky At Night* (Five Leaves 2003), *Smelter* (Mudfog 2003).

Chris Kinsey lives in Mid-Wales. She was awarded an Arts Council of Wales bursary in late 2000 and has written full time since. She either writes alone or with others in various settings. She has just become a Kung Fu instructor for Age Concern.

Mike Marqusee is an author and journalist. His books include *Anyone But England: Cricket and the National Malaise* (1994), *Redemption Song: Muhammad Ali and the Spirit of the Sixties* (1999) and *Chimes of Freedom: the Politics of Bob Dylan's Art* (autumn, 2003).

Biographies

Jay Merill lives in London. She has had stories published in quite a few literary magazines and has adapted one as a literary monologue which was performed in 2001 at the Lost Theatre One Act Festival in Fulham. Jay has currently just finished writing a novel. She is editorial assistant on *The London Magazine*.

Joan Michelson's chapbook *Letting in the Light* was the Editor's Choice 2002 Competition Winner Poeticmatrix Press CA, USA, available from poeticmatrix@yahoo.com. During the spring of 2003, she was a writing fellow in residence at Fundacion Valparaiso, Spain. She teaches creative writing at Birkbeck College, University of London.

Lee Morris was born in 1967 at Shoreham-by-Sea, Sussex. She spent her school-age years in South Aftrica, and returned to England to study music at the now Anglia Polytechnic University. She is at the moment a full-time mother to Luc (fivc) and Maia (one) and lives in Derbyshire.

Kathryn Moss was brought up in Basildon and now lives in Maidstone with her partner and son. She read English at Cambridge, but it took a National Extension College creative writing course to reconnect her with her childhood impulse to write poems. She works for House of Commons Hansard.

Daphne Rance lives in Baldock, Hertfordshire. "Living is the apprenticeship for writing: green growth and the blue of far horizons, red of pain, black despair. The hug of children, baking smells, flowers. Voices that delineate fellow people. Wonder. Choices that define oneself. These," says Daphne Rance, "are more important than what she did or where or when."

Noreen Rees was born within sight of the shipyards in Newcastle and now lives at the coast at Whitley Bay. In 2001 she won the People's Play award and later wrote the Passion Play for Whitley Bay so was responsible for closing the town centre to traffic for a day. Noreen is a member of Cloud Nine Theatre Company. She has an MA in Creative Writing from Northumbria and this is her second Biscuit.

Maurice Ryan is a Graduate in Greek and Latin Literature, Oxford University. Learned short story writing with the London School of Journalism. Later specialized in novel writing with the Leeds based *Writers' News*. Has spent the last 20 years as a lecturer of English overseas, including Poland, Kuwait, Saudi Arabia, United Arab Emirates and Borneo in South East Asia. Spends a lot of time in the Philippines where his wife comes from. Published *Studying in Britain*, a guide for overseas students in the UK. Currently publishing a full-length novel.

Leonie Smith, 28, resides in Suffolk. Now that she's finally got a story published, her only unfulfilled ambition is to be the first humorist on Mars. She'd aim for the Moon, but that joker Buzz Aldrin got there first.

David Swann was born four doors up from Jeanette Winterson, who

Biographies

polished her narrative craft by telling him ghost stories. Later he covered Accrington Stanley's even more frightening matches for the local rag. After working in Amsterdam, he became writer-in-residence at Nottingham Prison. He now teaches at University College, Chichester.

Elizabeth Tate was born and educated in the North of England. She is a practising artist and lectures in the Fine Art Department of Sunderland University. Her work is ideas led and covers a wide variety of materials and processes from text-based works to permanent site-related sculpture. She has exhibited widely, both nationally and internationally, and lives in Co. Durham with her dog and two horses.

Chris Turner began writing after joining Congleton Writers' Forum. He has had several short stories published in various anthologies and this makes his second entry in the 'Biscuit Top Twenty.' A chef by trade Chris is currently seeking a publisher for his collection of short stories covering the history of a mythical Arizona town.

Sue Vickerman's poetry pamphlet *Shag* will be published by Arrowhead in late 2003. Recently awarded £2000 from Arts Council of Scotland. Her poems and stories have appeared in many magazines and anthologies. A Yorkshire Arts Grant supported her short story collection *The Difference between Mark and Melissa*. Work-in-progress includes a novel *Special Needs*, and a full-length poetry collection for Biscuit. Sue lives in a lighthouse near Aberdeen.

Stephen Wade is a freelance writer and teacher. He has published over thirty short stories and also had several broadcast on local and national radio. His latest books are *WordShops* (Alphard) and *Somewhere Else* (Mellen, New York). He also writes True Crime and has just completed a book on murder cases in Calderdale.

Fay Wentworth has pursued her love of creative writing through a career, marriage and motherhood, and her stories have been published in children's and women's magazines. Recently changing direction, she took a home study course in mainstream fiction and is enjoying entering competitions and exploring new markets.

Sue Wood writes poetry and short stories, was a winner in 2002 Poetry Business Book and Pamphlet Competition with *Woman Scouring a Pot* (Smith/Doorstop) and has been placed in numerous other competitions for her poetry and stories. She runs writing workshops and is an occasional writer for "Alive and Kicking" Theatre Company based in Leeds. She has recently had one of her stories, *My Mum's a Slapper*, broadcast and put on a CD by the BBC.

Sally Zigmond has been writing seriously for over ten years. Her short fiction has been widely published and successful in major short-story competitions. She is the assistant editor of *QWF* magazine. She is writing her third novel with fingers crossed. She is married with two grown-up sons and lives in Yorkshire.